What a lesbian looks like

What a Lesbian Looks Like reflects the diversity of lesbian life in Britain today. Drawing on the mass-observation material of the National Lesbian and Gay Survey, it gives us glimpses into the lives and lifestyles of over fifty women of differing backgrounds and ideologies, and creates an impressionistic picture of a community seldom voluble about its private life.

The accounts were mainly written in response to a directive about each participant's earliest perceptions of lesbianism and coming to terms with her own sexuality. Where one woman might have been convinced of her sexuality from the age of seven, another might have no clear perception of the true nature of her sexuality until well into her thirties and forties. One writes of the natural attraction to a schoolfriend, another of discovering the joys of being a lesbian while in the armed forces, and another describes the distress she experienced at finding herself part of a despised minority. Though some had early negative experiences, the majority of women contributing to *What a Lesbian Looks Like* have transformed their lives, enabling themselves to pursue a positive lifestyle living with and relating to other women.

Written on a very personal level by the women involved, *What a Lesbian Looks Like* has a wide appeal, providing an inspiration to other lesbians of all ages. Rich in observation and memory, it is a fascinating compilation of lesbian life and experience today.

What a lesbian looks like

Writings by lesbians on their lives and lifestyles from the archives of the

National Lesbian and Gay Survey

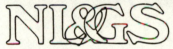

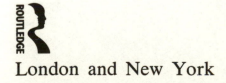

London and New York

First published in 1992 by
Routledge
11 New Fetter Lane, London EC4P 4EE

Simultaneously published in the USA and Canada
by Routledge
a division of Routledge, Chapman and Hall Inc.
29 West 35th Street, New York, NY 10001

Phototypeset by Intype, London
Printed and bound in Great Britain by
Mackays of Chatham PLC, Kent

British Library Cataloguing in Publication Data
A catalogue record for this book is available from the British Library

Library of Congress Cataloging in Publication Data
What a lesbian looks like: writings by lesbians and their lives and
    lifestyles/National Lesbian and Gay Survey.
    p.   cm.
    1. Lesbians—Great Britain. 2. Lesbianism—Great Britain.
    I. National Lesbian and Gay Survey (Organization)
    HQ75.6.G7W45   1992
    305.48'9664—dc20   91–43721
                                                                  CIP

ISBN 0–415–08155–6
        0–415–08100–9 (pbk)

Contents

National Lesbian and Gay Survey

During the 1930s a group of academics attempted to record the feelings and opinions of the person in the street on major issues of the day. Since then Mass-Observation has undergone many vicissitudes due largely to funding, or the lack of it, until it was formalized into a major national project and run from the University of Sussex.

My own involvement with the project began in the early 1980s. Each submission I made was chased up by a handwritten postcard from David Pocock, M-O's prime mover at the time, urging me on. It soon became clear that openly homosexual contributors were thin on the ground. An idea began to burgeon and, in the late summer of 1985, I set up the National Lesbian and Gay Survey in order to redress the balance. Since then lesbian and gay volunteers nationwide have written and submitted reports on a wide range of issues pertinent to lesbian and gay life.

The aims of the project are primarily archival, so that researchers of the future might understand what it was like to live as a homosexual in the late twentieth century. However, it has become clear that because the collection is rich in observation and memory much of it will be of interest to the reader today. It is that thought which led to this present anthology.

I would first of all like to acknowledge the important part played by Professor Pocock in the inspiration he provided during the setting up of the project, and to Dorothy Sheridan who is continuing his sterling work my thanks for her solidarity. I was a working volunteer and a director of the Hall-Carpenter Archives at the time and it was under the auspices of the Archives that NL&GS operated during its early years. I would like to acknowledge the support and encouragement of Julian Meldrum, the

Archives' founder, who first drew me into lesbian and gay archiving, and to the Archives' management team, particularly Peter Daniels, Margot Farnham, Oliver Merrington, David Stewart and Matthew Tagney. Thanks must also go to Kate Wilkinson, my co-director from 1985 to 1988, particularly for her input into the creation of directives.

On behalf of Kerry Sutton-Spence, currently the survey's Women's Director, and myself I would like to acknowledge the encouragement provided by our management group: Steven Barclay, Mandy Hagan, Duncan McDuffie, Raymond Parkes and Rachel Sutton-Spence. An enormous debt of gratitude must go to Michael Schofield for his financial generosity which has led to our being able to place and maintain a copy of the collection at the Mass-Observation Library at Sussex, together with a further copy available to researchers in Bristol. It is hoped that funds can be raised to provide further copies of the collection for researchers in Scotland, Northern Ireland, North Wales and the North-East of England. In the meantime, NL&GS continues its work with quarterly directives to an ever-increasing group of volunteers. This book does not mark the end of a project – it is very much part of the work in progress.

Kenneth Barrow
Founder, Men's Director

Introduction

NL&GS observers receive a quarterly directive. This is not a questionnaire but rather a series of suggestions of areas the volunteer might care to cover within a given topic. Directives are broad-based and try to approach the subject from every angle. In constructing a directive we are aware that sometimes we are being controversial, sometimes provocative and, occasionally, acting as devil's advocate.

The breadth of directives is matched by the diversity of the views expressed in the observers' written reports. Naturally, reports come in which take stances and express opinions quite alien to my own. But there is no censorship within NL&GS; everything submitted is logged and placed in the collection. Far too much of lesbian and gay history has previously been censored. In putting together this anthology we have attempted to reflect this diversity. There are conflicting views, there are contradictions. We make no attempt to draw conclusions, that is the prerogative of the readership whose views will be quite as diverse.

Because we have no control over the structure of the reports or of their content, they do not easily fall into preordained categories. The book is divided into nine parts. Sometimes it may seem that some of the extracts are rather arbitrarily grouped together. However, we have attempted to make the material as assimilable as possible.

All submissions made to NL&GS are entirely anonymous. As a result we are unable to credit any of the extracts to any individual. In order to make them more accessible and to identify serial submissions each author has been allocated a *nom de plume*. Observers are instructed to avoid the inclusion of circumstantial details and the naming of individuals. Where such was included in the original report, the circumstantial information has been removed and the names changed. The reasons behind this are that there are at least two sides to every story. What might constitute the truth to one might be claimed to be a libel by the other.

Lengthy reports have sometimes been shortened to avoid the unnecessary repetition of common areas of experience. Occasionally, a single paragraph has been isolated because of its particular relevance to that section's theme. Otherwise, apart from minor editing, the material appears here as it was submitted.

The oldest contributor to this anthology is in her sixties, the youngest was twenty when she first wrote a report to us. These women were mainly born in these islands, others come from Australia, America and Africa. They now live in Scotland, England and Wales. Some left school early, others have gone on to further education. There are unwaged women and those in high-powered jobs. The single thing they have in common is that they all identify as lesbian; well, with the proviso set out by Grace on page 143!

On behalf of NL&GS I would like to thank not only the authors of the work included in this volume, but all our volunteers for their sheer hard work in making this a vital and worthwhile collection.

Kerry Sutton-Spence
Women's Director

A month before I was due to leave the village, Maureen and I became lovers after a long talk one evening. Before this, I had never felt entirely at ease with her.

'It's wonderful,' I told my diary, 'to be open to feelings and emotions. I feel very opened up, like a horse whose blinkers have been removed.

'Catching a rare full-length view of myself in the mirror at the pub, I think – is this what a lesbian looks like?'

Susan

1

Beginnings

HELEN

I thought I was the only person in the world who loved her own sex. Even at seven I suspected my feelings were unusual. This must have been the case because I didn't tell anyone about them – not my mother or father, my sisters or my grandparents and certainly not the teachers and family friends I had fallen in love with. One would have thought that knowing I had to keep my feelings quiet would make me hate or suppress them, but my love for women made me happy. I remember at the age of eight hoping very much that when I grew up I wouldn't lose my passion for kind and beautiful women. I knew that most people (it felt like all people at the time) would be angry about my feelings – but I had a strong sense that, whatever anyone else thought, I was glad to love women. I didn't really care if they thought it was good or bad.

In some families all the men are farmers or pastry-makers. In my family all the men are psychiatrists. At the age of twelve I realized that their job was to 'treat' people like me – or, at least, people like me once they had grown up. I knew from overhearing some of their conversations that there were thoroughly sick people in the world who loved their own sex, men and sometimes women who wanted nothing better than to kiss each other and sleep in the same beds. It was very depressing to hear them speak like that. I didn't take their ideas on board, however. I thought, 'How shocking that these men have been pretending to be intelligent but are really so stupid.'

I felt angry with them – why couldn't they see how mean they were being? I knew in the back of my head that they were talking about the sort of person I would become – a homosexual.

My father's house was full of books about 'deviant personalities'. I started reading them when I was fourteen. It was all stuff like 'these people are immature and miserable – they will never be happy. Even if you see them cartwheeling across the road they are really covering up a profound resignation and despair'.

It was a revelation that the adult and academic world was really built upon personal opinion. Anyone on the inside of those feelings could tell at a glance. But in an odd sort of way it was still quite thrilling to read all these case histories. I hadn't found any lesbian novels yet; if I had I wouldn't have been reading case histories.

At school I was very isolated. This was the case throughout my school-days but it escalated as I got older. It never felt safe to show my real feelings. Even the grooviest, most left-wing girls at school expressed disdain and hatred towards gay people, who they invariably called 'queers'. If any of them went through a 'homosexual phase' they kept it well hidden. I suppose they must have; they are probably lesbians now, but most straight people are so terrified of 'abnormality' they would never have acknowledged any homosexual feelings. If they had it would have spelt instant humiliation and bullying.

When I was fourteen a lodger moved into our house. She was a feminist and the first out lesbian I ever met. I think my father was horrified by her. At mealtimes he would look at her badges and say things like, 'Oh, so you've gone off men, have you?' and kind of shrink into himself like he was under some sort of threat. I wanted her to fall in love with me so we could run away together. I thought she was such a cool, beautiful woman. I wanted to be like her more than anything else in the world. But I was young and boring and she hardly ever noticed me even though I followed her round the house and stared at her a lot.

When she moved away I thought, 'That's it, I'll never meet another lesbian again', as if they were so thin on the ground she was the only one who would ever cross my path. In fact, I wasn't too wrong, out lesbians were very rare at school. After her the first gay person I encountered was my new 'best friend' who I'd met in the co-ed sixth form. I didn't know he was gay when I first met him, but I did think it was strange I was getting on so

well with a boy. Of the two of us he was the first to 'confess'
he was gay. Shortly after that I admitted I was a lesbian.

Everyone thought we were going out together, including both
sets of parents. This was quite flattering for me because loads of
girls had crushes on him, but at the same time I didn't really like
people thinking I was straight.

When I was sixteen I fell into a deep depression. A woman
who I thought was clever and wonderful took me under her wing
and started counselling me. I'd been in love with her for a couple
of years before then. Maybe she knew it; maybe it gave her
power. I think she was probably a lesbian, but she was also a
Christian fundamentalist. I overlooked her religious extremism,
which was a very bad move, but she was the only person who
offered me any kind of support.

I never told her I was a lesbian. I thought she would just
somehow know. I wanted her to say, 'It's fine – I am, too!' but
one day she let it slip that her notion of counselling success would
be if I could 'get married and have children', as if that was the
summit of human happiness. I winced as she said those words.
I thought, 'Well, you have done none of these things yourself –
why are you telling me to do them?'

In retrospect I can see that no heterosexual ever helped me to
come to terms with my sexuality. Ninety per cent of them tried
to hinder it – not always directly (because they didn't necessarily
know I was a lesbian) but their attitudes always implied a hatred
of homosexuality. The media didn't help much either. When I
was quite young an MP was 'exposed' and hounded by the press
for her lesbianism. My stepmother said, 'It's disgusting, she lives
with another woman as if they were married and everything.' I
saw this woman's face on television. She looked like a perfectly
pleasant person. I hated the way she was being treated, as if she
were a murderer or something. I cannot remember her name,
but I have never forgotten her face, which is interesting because
I really was very young at the time. I have a photographic
memory for faces, maybe because as a young lesbian homosexuality was very rarely spoken about. Their faces expressed
more than their words. I had to look very carefully at them to
see how they really felt.

My best friend and I started to go to gay clubs together. I
would have preferred to visit women-only places, but I was shy
and I liked what's-his-face. During one of our forays into the

gay world I did eventually make friends with another woman. I was eighteen, she was about five years older than me. I was profoundly amazed that she was interested in me and, without much thought, fell into a relationship with her.

The first time we slept together I was overwhelmed. Physical closeness to another person, any other person, was completely outside my experience. I think I had a sort of small breakdown. I felt as if I was disintegrating. This was, in some part, due to my lover's sudden revelation of her Catholicism. In her opinion our relationship was evil. She said she had told a priest about it and he had warned her it was a cardinal sin. After that she announced we had to split up.

This was 1983 in inner London at the height of the GLC's so-called campaign to 'promote homosexuality'. Where were the 'positive images', the 'pro-gay propaganda'? If it ever existed I never saw any and my first lover certainly didn't. She could have done with it – she tried to commit suicide more than once.

I think I was luckier than her. My parents are both atheists and they never pushed any notions of 'sin' or 'evil' upon their children, though they both have their fair share of secular bigotry and dogmatism. At least I escaped religious guilt. I came out to my parents when I was eighteen. I didn't stand up in the middle of their sitting-room and shout, 'Listen here, everybody – I'm a lesbian!' I just never told any lies or covered anything up. I let them know the woman I was living with was my lover. I think they probably knew I was a lesbian before that, though. When I was fourteen I'd cropped my hair and announced I was a feminist. I was always going on about how superior I thought women were. Their reaction to my lesbianism was very bland and reticent. At least they didn't say 'you are disgusting and a pervert', but by then I'd been thrown out of home for other reasons and they knew I didn't care what straight people thought.

CATHY

My middle school in Leeds was rough and the kids largely working class and it was common for the words 'lez' or 'lezzie' to be used as terms of abuse by both girls and boys. I knew this meant some female who had a dirty attitude towards, or involvement with, other women. It was a really contemptuous word to use and I remember feeling sorry for a girl called Lesley because someone might realize that she could be nicknamed 'Les' and start teasing her. I couldn't understand how parents could choose such a name! I can't remember anyone ever explaining homosexuality to me at that stage but have some vague memories of seeing *Tom Brown's Schooldays* on television and associating boys' schools with odd behaviour in bedrooms. But it certainly wasn't as bad as being called a 'lezzie'. That attitude to lesbians remained right through until my first year in the sixth form when I was stung and humiliated by a drunken lad suggesting that my best friend and I were 'lesbians' because I insisted on waiting for her to go home with. But by then the feeling of having been insulted had little connection with my inner and more positively developing ideas about my attraction to women.

TANYA

I remember being on a school holiday at the age of thirteen and chasing a schoolfriend around the hotel room when she had only her underwear on. This was a very embarrassing memory for me for a long time, although she never mentioned it again and we were friends for a long time afterwards.

At the time I didn't feel homosexual. It was more that I perceived myself as male. I dressed in boys' clothes and was brought up very much with boys, including my brother, until I went to an all-girl convent school at the age of eight. I didn't begin to perceive myself as a girl until I was about fourteen. I remember looking at myself in the mirror and realizing that I had been seeing myself as something I wasn't.

My brother once asked my mother how she would feel if one of her children was gay (this must have been when I was about seventeen). She said, 'Don't be silly' but when pressed she said that it would be very sad. I remember feeling uncomfortable and wishing the conversation would end. Homosexuality was often talked about in the family in a jokey sort of way. I don't remember it being talked about at school. I imagine that I was presented with negative images since it is only now, at the age of twenty-four, with four years of more or less conscious lesbianism behind me, that I have made some headway about feeling positive about it.

JESSICA

There was a programme on television one evening. I must have been about eight. In it a woman declared herself a lesbian and spoke of her feelings for women. I didn't understand most of the discussion, but I remember knowing - somehow - that this 'lesbian', whatever it was, somehow related to the way I felt. I remember being a bit scared. However unintelligible the language, the tone of the programme was very clear in its disapproval. I determined to keep this moment of self-discovery to myself until I felt sure of my ground.

So, at the age of eight or nine, I had the terminology; certainly by the time I was eleven words like 'poof' and 'lez' were bandied about the playground as general terms of abuse for anyone who didn't fit the accepted criteria, but I doubt if anyone truly knew what they meant.

Somewhere along the line between then and meeting the first openly gay person I knew, I gleaned a little more information, but from where I cannot recall. The subject was never discussed at home; there were no visibly gay characters in the books I read and I don't remember any other television programmes devoted to the subject. In retrospect I think I was a little afraid to find out. If you're tentative about who you are, anyway, you don't make waves by aligning yourself with 'unacceptable' minorities.

I'd always felt quite 'different' as a child, although I could never pinpoint for why. For a long time I believed I should have been born a boy because I felt very uneasy in typically feminine roles. Being made to wear a dress and 'play nicely' was torture; I was happiest up a tree with dirty knees and holes in my shorts. Not that I was actively discouraged from being a boisterous girl child, I simply felt an unspoken expectation for me to grow out of it and an innate knowledge that I couldn't.

I'd also always had strong feelings towards women. Again, in retrospect, I feel that this was the root of my belief I should really have been a boy. Had I been male I could have expressed my interest in the girls around me. As it was, I knew I should keep quiet about it. I felt there was something 'wrong' about these feelings, but could never quite fathom quite what, because it felt so natural. There were girls who were my friends and there were girls for whom I had 'special' feelings. As a child this was simply a desire for a closeness beyond that of our usual friendship, but as I grew older these feelings did not abate; instead they grew more intense. While not overtly sexual, they nevertheless craved a greater intimacy than simple friendship permitted.

Throughout this time I never once considered the possibility I might be gay. I think I was scared to – I still hadn't truly fathomed out what being gay was, except it was something no one wanted to be. The feelings I had for women were something secret and so long as they remained so I didn't need to deal with them. But I did become quite solitary as I went into my teens, afraid they might escape and expose me as something horrific. I remember being quite afraid of fortune-tellers or anyone vaguely mystic, for fear they would be able to recognize the Real Me. I was also afraid of getting too close to any of the women I liked in case I revealed an interest in them that they'd recognize. (I never considered what their recognition might reveal about them!)

Ironically enough, in the midst of all this hiding, from myself and everyone else, I also came out, to everyone except myself, in that my best friend and I had a huge and very public crush on our biology teacher, so all our class-mates began to think of us and refer to us as 'the lesbians', but without rancour. Still, I didn't relate this to my other secret feelings about women. It was a bit of a joke to have the hots for Ms Baker. To reveal you also fancy the girl in the next desk was a bit too much like real life, and might not have been received as well.

I trundled along in this confused fashion until I was sixteen. About that time I met Tony, a friend of a friend. He was the first openly gay man I'd met, and he scared me to death! He was extremely camp, very loud and shrill and, while I was fascinated by the entertainment value of his performance, I found his tales of cottaging and doing drag depressing. I wanted to be able to talk to him, to lay my emerging doubts about my own sexuality before him and find reassurance, but I didn't trust him to be sensible. I continued to see him, because I had a vague hope he might recognize my homosexuality and point me in the right direction, but I think he was having too much trouble dealing with his own to be able to help anyone else.

Daunted by this, and by trips I'd made with Tony and my friend to gay clubs, where everyone was intent on scoring to the detriment of anything else, I retreated back to the closet to lick my wounds. I still did not acknowledge I might be gay, I was just showing an interest in alternative lifestyles. It amazes me now how steadfastly I clung to this idea, even though the odds were mounting against me.

It took another year before I came out. I went to see a play called *Cloud Nine* which had several gay characters in it. Moreover, gay actors were playing the roles, so I felt more inclined to believe in the truth of their performance. The gay men and lesbians they portrayed were very real characters, not caricatures or perverse or miserable, just ordinary people with real lives that didn't revolve around toilets or clubs. I saw the show four or five times. Each time I felt better, safer for having spent that time in the company of characters I knew to be real. Finally, from that nest of security, I felt able to look inward and acknowledge my own homosexuality.

RUTH

Right from the age of seven, at primary school, I got crushes on older girls. I can even remember the names of two girls (older than me) who I liked or perhaps hero-worshipped at that age. I remember my mother telling me it was natural to have crushes on older girls and how she'd experienced that as a schoolgirl. Having a secure and loving family I didn't worry too much about my attachments to other girls. I never felt any hostility or antagonism towards boys; indeed, I was the proverbial tomboy in shorts and T-shirts, joining in with the boys in their games and gangs. It was just that my emotional attachments always seemed to be directed towards other girls. I think I was probably aware from a very early age of the strength of my feelings for members of the same sex. At the age of eight I was friendly with a girl of eleven. One day at her house she suggested we both take all our clothes off and pretend to be grown-ups who were married. I did as she suggested but didn't enjoy the feeling very much. I remember thinking what we were doing wasn't 'normal' and she was much more enthusiastic about it than I was. She didn't assault me and nothing horrible happened but I felt guilty afterwards. She moved up to senior school and we rarely saw each other afterwards.

At the age of ten or eleven I developed a particularly strong crush on one of the girls in my class. We became best friends and would sometimes kiss each other on the mouth. I remember liking the feeling of her being so close to me. It was always incorporated somehow in a game we played but I gradually became bored with the game and felt I'd like to get straight to the part where I touched her and kissed her. That stopped after about a year.

As I became an adolescent and more aware of what my sexuality meant, I tended to ignore it. I started going out with boys at fourteen and continued to do so on a fairly serious basis until I was about nineteen. All the time I was aware that my attraction to women was not diminishing and indeed was becoming stronger. But I felt isolated. I was growing up surrounded by heterosexuals and knew no other lesbians or gay men.

At seventeen I got a Saturday job and one of my fellow workers was a gay man about two years older than me. He was quite open about his sexuality and I felt thrilled to have at least met someone the same as me – even if he was the wrong sex! We never discussed my sexuality; I probably would have denied it if he'd asked me. Not having had a physical encounter with a member of my own sex since the age of eleven, I hardly felt I was a lesbian. Emotionally, I still felt attracted to women but physically I was a practising heterosexual.

Then another girl started working there. I was attracted to her and suspected she might be a lesbian. We became friendly and started to see each other outside work. For about two months we skirted around the issue until one night she admitted she was gay. God, I felt so happy! Here at last was a fellow spirit. It took another two weeks until one night I kissed her. This was confirmation of everything I'd ever felt – it felt so right to kiss another woman.

Unfortunately, the relationship floundered after about four months. I was paranoid about anyone finding out about us. I felt racked with guilt at someone bursting in through the door every time she so much as touched my arm. We never progressed beyond kissing, hugging and minor groping. I was too frightened to sleep with her – fear of my and her inexperience as much as fear of being discovered as a lesbian. Outside of her I knew no other lesbians. Everywhere I turned heterosexuality was the norm. My brother suspected my relationship and made some homophobic comments which made me even more scared and paranoid. I'm sure it's because, seeing no other manifestation of gay life or relationships, I didn't know where to look for help or encouragement. The sad thing is, how right it felt to hold her, and how that was mainly destroyed by fear and paranoia about other people's reactions and rejection.

DOROTHY

By the time I was thirteen, I thought I might be a lesbian. My strongest feelings were towards other women. I had been a heroine worshipper from an early age. (I recall, with a smile, my five-year-old fantasy of rescuing my teacher from a frozen death by clutching her to my chest and marching across the wastes of Antarctica to warmth and safety.) With the onset of puberty I started feeling lustful rather than admiringly awed. I knew of Freud's theory of the latent homosexual phase, so figured it might be something I would grow out of. I was, after all, incarcerated in an all-girls' school. But, at gut level, I felt it was for keeps, not merely the emotional equivalent of a training bra.

I first expressed my lesbian self at fifteen when I made a pass at one of my teachers. This didn't go down well. On finding out, my mother used her professional connections to get our family into therapy very fast with a shrink who was, without doubt, a dyke. Some irony there. Since I didn't want to be involved I did my damnedest to block it all out, and consequently lack memories of that period.

ISLA

I never connected either the medical descriptions I found in the text books and encyclopaedias in the library or the playground whispers with the feelings I had which I'd been aware of for some time. I didn't connect it with myself until whispers started at school that my best friend and I were lesbians. I was appalled at the suggestion. When people began to say it to our faces and to be abusive, threatening and finally violent, I went back to the library and read in earnest, but nothing seemed to describe me. I heard of a book called *The Well of Loneliness* and tried to borrow it from the library. I never succeeded. It was always out and I was afraid to request it as that meant giving my name and address and I was frightened the librarian would inform my parents.

My friend and I had known each other all our lives and had progressed from giving each other massages to sexual intimacy. I never thought of this as homosexual or us as homosexuals until other people labelled us with the term. Although my first homosexual sexual experience was satisfying physically it was otherwise very oppressive. My lover insisted on dead secrecy; no one was to know. She would never kiss me, although we made love. Eventually, I tentatively suggested to her that we *might* be lesbians. She hit me hard and told me never to use that word to her again. We were unique friends. Other people were homosexuals.

I still wasn't sure what a homosexual was. I loved women and I got a guilty thrill when homosexuality was mentioned or I read about it. But did that make me one? I didn't know where to turn.

The school informed my parents that they thought I was having an 'unnatural friendship' but they didn't take it seriously. The school suggested an educational psychologist and a care order but my parents refused to consider it. Not knowing that the reason I truanted from school was to escape harassment, they said all I needed was to be forced to attend. My lover left me as she couldn't stand the pressure at school.

Eventually, due to all this, I left school, home, town. My parents were still in blissful ignorance and couldn't understand why I wanted to leave. Once in the big city things improved. I met people who had no negative views about homosexuality, and met gay people through them. I told no one of my own feelings and experiences but I began to get positive images of gays and lesbians. I made gay and lesbian friends and through these friendships was introduced to the gay scene and to gay books and movies. I still refused to accept my own lesbianism but I began to confide in other gays who were supportive, sympathetic and patient. I shared a flat with a gay man who was wonderful. At the age of twenty-three I finally felt happy with my identity as a lesbian and came out and, for the first time, felt happy about sex.

MEG

When I was thirteen our family moved towns. I remember very clearly my first day at my new school. While the Principal was showing my parents and me round the school and singing its praises, a tall dark-haired girl interrupted him, carrying another girl who had just overdosed on tranquillizers. It was a great

advert for a school for me, but my parents were a little put out
to say the least!

I didn't even have the usual trauma of breaking into the scene
of the new school. Kelly, the dark-haired beauty, who was the
most popular girl in the school for her sporting abilities, her great
practical jokes and her open rebelliousness, for some reason really
took a shine to me and I was immediately made a member of
the 'inner clique'. Kelly and I became inseparable. We spent all
day together at school, even getting there earlier than necessary
in order to have more time together. After school, we spent
hours together until we would have to part reluctantly to go to
our homes. What did we find to talk about for all those hours?
Weekends we used to spend at each other's homes.

Neither of us could articulate it (not even to each other then)
but we knew that the physical attraction and the over-the-top
liking for each other was more than 'just friends'. At the time
there used to be a put-down which went 'Lez-be-friends'. We
were called this all the time, but it didn't sound so bad to me.
Eventually, after months of faking falls and faints, pretending to
sleep and dropping my arm out of bed so that she would gently
have to put it back, we kissed. Wow, what a kiss! Talk about
the earth moving! It was electrifying, and from that moment on
we were hot lovers, positively rampant! We used to go into the
girls' loos and get it off, but all in absolute silence. We became
masters of the Silent Fuck. Of course, we told no one at school
for fear of persecution.

My mum and dad used to work until about six o'clock, so
that meant we had a couple of hours' privacy to go to bed (after
I'd gotten rid of my little brother). A couple of times we got so
carried away we didn't hear mum come home and she walked in
on us, hard at it! Horror!! She reacted like her daughter was being
raped by the devil, banned Kelly from the house for ever, and
tried to make me feel vile, repulsive and sick. She did make me
feel terrible, mainly because I could see that this split between us
was irreparable, but I always knew deep down that the love and
care Kelly and I had for each other could never be an evil thing,
and that the badness was in my mother's head and in society's
attitude. However, we had *no one* else to turn to for support and
affirmation, we only had each other. In fact, my mother always
regarded me with suspicion from then on and I never forgave
her for her bigotry and narrow-mindedness, until the moment

before she died, when I allowed myself to forgive, for, after all, she was only the product of her background and conditioning.

I left home shortly after that, at the age of fifteen, on the pretext that it was too difficult for me to find work in a small country town. My real reason was to be with Kelly. We set up house together, with other friends (mixed) and Kelly and I lived together for a further six years in total subterfuge. Even though we were all supposedly liberated, seventies drug-taking, political rebels, Kelly and I still didn't feel safe enough to tell our friends about our relationship. We had a room together but with separate, single beds. I'm talking about the years 1969 to 1975 in Queensland, Australia, when we were still in the dark ages.

STEPH

I was aware of my feelings for a long time before I knew there was a name for them. In fact, long before I knew there was a name for anything! I was passionately in love with Julie Rogers when I was nine (she was a singer – of 'The Wedding' fame). These days I deplore my early taste, but then she was my dream. I had pin-up posters of her all over my half of the bedroom and I spent a considerable amount of time indulging in day-dreams, fantasizing how I would rescue her from some peril – kidnapping or terrorists or something – and she would faint gratefully in my arms, and then we'd live happily ever after. I was much too young and innocent to know what came between the fainting and the 'happy-ever-after' but whatever it was I was sure it was wonderful.

The next clear memory I have of any kind of emotions was some time between eleven and twelve in my first year of high school. I started getting the same feelings about a girl in my class, and putting her into the same kind of day-dreams. I knew enough by then to add a couple of kisses (no tongues!) before the happy-ever-after bit. I found myself trying to get her attention, to like me, showing off if I knew she was watching. I discovered I could make her laugh, so I became court jester for a while. Looking back, I'm sure she was having the same kind of feelings but didn't know what to do with them either. She's an actress now, and I know for a fact that she's bisexual. But, back then, I didn't know how she felt. I didn't care as long as I could be with her. It must've been fairly obvious that I had a crush on her. When I was twelve, right at the beginning of my second year, a couple of classmates passed by and one of them said, 'You know, if I was a lez, I'd go for Geraldine as well.' I didn't have any feelings about the phrase except curiosity; I'd never heard the word. I couldn't find 'lez' in the dictionary either. I went to Frankie, the class know-all, to see if she knew. After careful checking that no one was listening, she explained that 'lez' was short for lesbian and it meant women who went to bed with other women. I mulled over this for a while. 'What? You mean girls fall in love with girls like boys?' 'Yes,' she said. I said 'Thanks' and went away to digest this information. I couldn't see anything wrong with it. It seemed perfectly natural. I thought, 'Fine, I've got a name. I'm a lez.' It didn't bother me in the slightest and I promptly dismissed it from my mind, and carried on having crushes for the next couple of years on three or four more girls and a couple of teachers (French and Maths, to be precise. Our gym teacher was a vicious drill-sergeant who looked like the loser in a head-butting contest with a steam train!).

At fifteen the word was brought to my attention again. By this time my best friend, and subject of my current crush, was Felicity – masses of wavy auburn hair, blue eyes – and I thought she was marvellous. I had my own room now, not shared with my sister, and Janis Joplin and Joan Baez had replaced Julie Rogers on the wall. Felicity and I would often lock ourselves in and talk for hours after school about pop stars and films. In spite of being underaged we'd sneaked in to see both *The Graduate* and *Rosemary's Baby* during our afternoon 'playing hooky' sessions. Felicity thought Dustin Hoffman was the living 'It' – absolutely groovy – and we'd talk about boyfriends, not that either of us had ever had one, but it was expected that we would talk about them, and make an effort to acquire one soon. Personally, I wasn't bothered. I had absolutely no interest whatsoever in boys.

One afternoon – for some reason I remember quite clearly that it was a Wednesday – we were lying on the bed, as usual, propped up on our elbows when Felicity asked me if I'd ever been kissed. When I said I hadn't she confessed that neither had she, and then suggested that perhaps we ought to get some practice. After all, boys would think we were silly if we'd no idea how to kiss them. Being unbelievably thick I asked how we were supposed to do that. She said we could practise with each other, and promptly suited the action with words. My God, did she know how to kiss. Every afternoon from then on we'd go home and practise kissing for hours. I discovered tongues! This went on for about three months, nothing more than kissing, though I discovered that, sometimes, kissing started feelings in other places. I didn't quite know what to do with that.

Then we got careless. A quick kiss snatched in the loo while sneaking a cigarette, or in the changing-room at the gym – sooner or later we were bound to get caught. Not that I knew why we were hiding or why I wasn't supposed to tell anyone. It all seemed perfectly natural to me. The crunch came when my mother received an anonymous letter, as did Felicity's, from someone at school, calling us perverts and so on. It was quite a nasty, sick letter from what little I remember. Mum flipped, asked if it was true, and then blew her top. I was grounded for a couple of weeks, and kept away from school. When I returned I found that Felicity's parents had taken her away from the school completely. I went round to see her. She wouldn't take the door off the chain. She told me I was a filthy pervert, sick, that I'd corrupted her, that it was all my fault, that I was a nasty lezzie, and that she never wanted to see me again. At which point her mother came home, said roughly the same things and threatened to call the police. Her mother called my mother on a neighbour's phone, as we didn't have one of our own. By the time I got home my mother was on the warpath. She told me she was going to tell my dad when he came back at the weekend. I knew what the reaction would be and I didn't fancy getting the living daylights beaten out of me. I ran away from home. The police brought me back four days later.

When I got back to school the fun really started. There had always been whispers about me, but mostly good-natured jokes about keeping my hands in sight or who was sharing my room on school trips. The good-natured jokes stopped and things got nasty. No one would sit near me, and at recess and lunch-breaks and my other free time before and after school, the gang of girls who considered themselves the toughest, about ten or twelve of them, would follow me everywhere I went, chanting 'lezzie, lezzie' or asking questions about what I did and who with. (They had some fairly bizarre ideas of lesbian sex!) There would be messages in my desk; my coat and books mysteriously disappeared regularly, turning up in a puddle, or smothered in ink and the like. I stuck it out for a year, then I dropped out of school.

I'd thoroughly got the message though. I was sick, perverted, disgusting and no decent person would associate with me. I started to acquire a deep self-hatred and a sense of shame. I withdrew totally into myself. I had always been a bit of a tomboy, but now I had got the message – lesbians were imitation men. I became *very* butch.

My mother took me to the doctor when I was sixteen after collapsing with asthma. He took her aside to discuss my 'problem' and suggested hormone shots! My mother became very indignant, and we all changed our doctor. She had never told my father. I didn't realize it then, but she probably knew all about me and accepted me, but didn't know how to tell me it was okay.

Just before my fourteenth birthday I saw my first ever lesbian in the media – Shirley Maclaine in a movie called *The Loudest Whisper.*★ It was on as the late-night movie on BBC2. In the end she commits suicide. After it, to my complete surprise, I burst into tears. I'm not sure why – the previous two years of hell, shame and guilt, I expect. Over the next couple of years I saw a couple more movies and television shows, and I found *The Well of Loneliness*. The message was the same each time. There was a 'real' lesbian, generally mannish, though not always, and a 'real' woman who eventually left the lesbian, usually for a man. The lesbian then committed suicide, conveniently. She was always a sad, pathetic figure, or totally despised and unlikeable. I was getting the message loud and clear by now. That year my family left London to live in the West Country. That large cathedral city proved to be just as forward-thinking and tolerant as I expected. It was 1972, there was a gay movement, things were happening, but it might as well have been on the dark side of the moon for all the information I had. Then I discovered alcohol. It didn't make anything better, but sometimes it could make you forget the hurt.

Then something good happened, for a change. I discovered a real lesbian – *another one*! She was thirty-four and married with two sons. I was seventeen and ignorant. It was only a one-night stand, but what a night. I learned an incredible amount, almost enough to show me how ignorant I really was. But, at last, I finally knew, yes, sex with a woman was fantastic. It was right.

★ British title of *The Children's Hour* (1961) from Lillian Hellman's play of the same name.

It was natural. There was no alternative. This was who I was. It was an action-packed year. I became fairly promiscuous (when I could find other dykes!), my father died, and I was rapidly disappearing into a bottle.

The year 1974 came. I was nineteen and another great thing happened. I discovered *Gay News* and *Sappho*. They rapidly became my lifeline. There were *loads* of others out there and they weren't unhappy, they were glad and proud. By now I'd had so much practice at self-hating that this seemed like a revolutionary concept. Then I fell in love. She was straight. She didn't believe me, but we stayed friends. I decided to tell my mother. It was hardly a proud coming out. I got drunk and cried a lot and told her I was 'queer'. She said – and I remember her words exactly – 'Yes, of course you are, dear. Now pop the kettle on and let's have a nice cup of tea.' I have never sobered up so fast in my life. She completely and totally accepted it and always has. She invited me home for Christmas with my girlfriend, referred to herself as my friend's 'mother-in-law' and accepts any change in partner or lifestyle with a completely unruffled attitude that still sometimes leaves me gasping, especially when I see the trouble some others have with their parents.

In early 1975 my friend finally believed me and decided she might be in love with me too, although she was still certain she wasn't gay, and we moved in together. She pulled me firmly out of the bottle. The only real problem with our relationship was that I spent our entire time together just waiting for her to run off with a man. She got totally fed up with this expectation and did.

I had now decided I was gay and proud of it. I started wearing badges, going on marches and talking about it to anyone who would listen. I was twenty, but I wasn't really 'proud'. I hadn't really accepted it myself. Oh, I don't mean I thought there was any alternative. There wasn't. I couldn't be anything other than gay, but I still wasn't (for want of a better word) comfortable with it. I was loud, pushy, aggressive and defensive.

My lover had returned. Throughout our time together she would, infrequently, get involved with a man before returning to me. She had a lot of parent trouble and took a long time to come to terms with her sexuality. She wasn't as lucky as me; she did have the alternative and it confused her.

Some time, around age twenty-six or seven, I started to realize

I didn't need to be pushy any more. If somebody asked, I would tell them, or if it came up in conversation, or if I needed to correct any anti-gay remark or joke, but I wasn't being aggressive any more. The defensiveness has gone. I seem to have developed what I call 'quiet acceptance'. I think that I have finally come to terms with my sexuality properly.

My feelings now are that I love being a woman. I love being a lesbian; I wouldn't change it if I could. I love women and making love with women. I'm back to being fairly promiscuous again. I find that if I'm in a serious relationship I'm faithful, and I work hard at it, but if I'm not in a 'proper' relationship I tend to have a few, three or four continuing but casual affairs. I don't go in for one-night stands much, but I wouldn't object if someone I liked really wanted one! If people can't handle that – too bad, but life's too short to worry about them. I give all my energy to the people I care about. I don't have any time for people who disapprove or think I'm sick. There are still people like that.

To borrow a Kylie Minogue song title – yes, we play some tacky music at our discos too! – 'I wouldn't change a thing'. My adolescence was no picnic, but if I hadn't gone through that then, maybe, I wouldn't be as happy now.

2

Kin

SARA

I grew up in the very liberal setting of an artists' community in Cornwall. There was a great deal of tolerance of homosexuality, on the whole, and I have memories of there always being gay men around. My mother had, and still has, many gay men friends and, as a teenager, I stayed with them in London, and they stayed with us at home. My father wasn't at all happy about Mum's friends and blamed the break-up of their marriage on a woman friend of my mother's. In fact, he was having a lot of affairs and leaving all the bringing up of my brother and me to my mother. He left to live in London when I was about fourteen. My mother's friend lived with us and shared her bedroom. However, it wasn't until I was around thirty and thinking about my own sexuality, that I realized that this was a lesbian relationship. I have been able to talk to my mother and her friend about this as they are still friends, spending each Sunday together. She was like an older sister to me and is in Mum's will, the same as my brother and I. This is fine by me. She must have been so supportive to my mother at a very difficult time in my mother's life. She has relationships with men now. As far as I know my mother has not had any other relationships since with either sex.

JUDY

When I was getting used to the idea that I was a lesbian and beginning to make friends on the gay scene, I had my first physical sexual experience with another woman. It was not actu-ally very good at all as both of us had been drinking and, for my part, there was no real sexual attraction to this woman, but I was not sure how to refuse her and felt it was something I *had* to do – almost just to get it over with! My next sexual partner was a woman I lived with for five years but I couldn't honestly say that even then the sex was good. My partner did not (and does not) enjoy sexual intimacy. We have now separated but she has not settled with any other partner either in terms of sexual compatibility. At the time we were together I felt very badly about my sexual appetite and desires as she disliked that side of things. It wasn't until I had a brief encounter with a woman who 'picked me up' on the tube in London and took me back to her place, that I had a happy sexual experience. She was as passionate about sex as I am and we had uninhibited and pleasurable sex in the week we were together.

I had confided my sexuality to my mother after I became involved in my first lesbian relationship and she just said that she already suspected as much . . . and that was all. She was neither positive nor negative about it and didn't seem to want to talk so I was not able to discuss that part of my life with her. Four years after I came out my mother separated from my dad and, subsequently, started a lesbian relationship with a work colleague. She did not, at first, let anyone else in the family know until I asked her about her 'friendship'. Since then, she and her girlfriend have been living together and are both very happy. My youngest sister also came out in her late teens. As I am the oldest child in our family, and my sister had also seen my mum settle down with another woman, it was probably easier for her to come to terms with her sexuality than it was for me, having no role models or even knowledge of lesbianism as a child. My mother does not consider that she was always lesbian and said she enjoyed her marriage to my dad while it lasted – approximately thirty years – but she now identifies as lesbian in her present relationship.

PAULA

My best friend was the girl next door. Carrie was the same age as me. One of the games we played when we were about ten or twelve years old involved us hugging and holding each other. At the time, I knew that I enjoyed that game, and that it felt different and pleasurable. I did not then recognize those feelings as sexual.

Later, when I experienced sexual arousal and understood what it was, I remembered those games and reinterpreted the feelings they aroused in me.

At the time of my friendship with Carrie, my mother asked me one day what she and I did when we played in her bedroom. Even though I felt innocent of any wrongdoing, and believed my friendship and games with Carrie to be totally good and acceptable, I knew there was trouble looming with my mother, so I lied. I did not tell her about the hugging and holding game, because I knew she would say it was wrong and sick. Even so, she forbade me to play inside with Carrie unless the weather was so bad that we could not play outside, and she made it clear that anything Carrie and I did in her bedroom must be wrong and abnormal and disgusting.

My sister, Julia, is a lesbian and lived with the same woman from the age of eighteen till she was forty. However, I did not allow myself to know she was a lesbian until I was about thirty. My father asked me, when I was eighteen, if I thought Julia and the woman she lived with were lesbians. I replied that I did not know, and that it was none of my business anyway. I think that at the time I thought they were lesbians, and that I was protecting them. I believe that, as my politics and my friendship with women developed, I refused to believe that Julia and the woman she lived with could be lesbians, as that would have challenged my own position.

When I was a child, we had two friends, Miss Ashton and Miss Carpenter. Miss Ashton was twenty years younger than Miss Carpenter and took care of her. They lived together, and I remember that I was interested in the fact that though they had two bedrooms they shared one of them, leaving the other empty. As I got into my teens, I began to believe that they were lesbians (or whatever my vocabulary allowed me to think), and that was fine by me.

When I was sixteen, I began to be involved in the local repertory theatre, and I soon realized that some of the men were homosexual. They, and everyone in the theatre, were completely open about it and, as everyone showed that it was okay, and as I was continuing to rebel against my parents' views, I had no antipathy towards them. Indeed, the kindness and friendliness shown by some of them probably helped to shape my view that gay was okay. For others, though, not for me.

Paradoxical as it may seem, I am convinced that I finally reached the position where I dared to express the sexual feelings I had had for several years, because of the heterosexual relationship I was in at the time. When I was thirty-two I began what turned out to be the longest-lasting (two years), safest, most comfortable, least threatening relationship I ever had with a man. Till then I had been very unhappy, considering myself too unattractive, unloveable, tall, intellectual, feminist, anything, to have a 'normal' relationship with a man. I was never in a couple and never felt accepted by the straight world I inhabited. With this relationship came my acceptance of myself as a worthwhile human being. I believe that one of the reasons I was able to let go of my heterosexuality and seize my lesbianism with such enthusiasm and determination was because I felt good about myself for the first time in my adult life.

ELAINE

I live in two worlds. I'm not out at work or at home and I lead two separate lives. My friends at the sports club where I play don't really know, with the odd exceptions. My friend is the same age. We've been friends for sixteen years, quite close, and it was to her that I first admitted I was gay. This was not, however, until after I'd been seeing a man for quite a while and we/he decided that he wanted to live with me. I wanted this as well, not really because we were in love but we were good mates. We used to go out on his motor bike and do things like that together, and we both wanted to get away from our parents so we began to think about it. It was then we had rather a nasty accident on the motor bike and I was quite badly injured. He came to see me every day as he had only slight injuries. When I came out of hospital he came twenty miles a day to see me even though I knew it was a chore for him, but it was the highlight of my day because he could take me out and I'd had to sit indoors most of the day. It was two and a half to three years before I could move about again and we found a place to live and set up home. My parents, who are very archaic, were pleased in one way, that I was living with a man, but they wanted us to marry. We were very happy. Sex wasn't very good, but I thought that was just me. Occasionally, I used to lie in bed and cry but I didn't know why. Jeff used to get upset too. Eventually, I started going to see a therapist about the sex problem and she was so good. I was only meant to see her a couple of times but I ended up going to see her for a year and a half.

I think she knew I was gay from the beginning but she never said; she let me talk it out. Gradually, though, I began to feel like a balloon that is being blown up until I was ready to burst. Jeff and I went on holiday. We had a nice time and came back on the Saturday morning. My sister, nine years younger than me, came to see me. I'd known she was gay for a few years, when I'd visited her flat (she'd been thrown out at home with these words from my father, 'I'd rather she'd been a prostitute'). When my sister came to visit me she asked for directions how to get to a place twenty miles away where there was a gay disco. On the spur of the moment I asked her to take me along. I lied that I'd been to that sort of place before and she was really shocked. So was I, really, but the more she backed down the more firm I was until she agreed. I'd never been to a disco before and I found it very loud. I was about twenty-seven then. When we got there I met a girl I used to work with and always fancied and she'd tried very hard to get to know me, but then I was on my 'straight kick'. She got quite drunk and, although she was with someone, she danced very provocatively with me. I didn't see her for a while after that but I'll always remember her. I still find her very attractive but she's settled down now.

Anyway, later that night I met a girl who danced the slow ones with me and I asked lots of, I thought, impertinent questions. She was very drunk but didn't appear to be. Her name was Valerie. She worked fairly near me and I saw her a few times in her place of work, until one day she asked me out. We went out together for a year until she met a girl who was supposedly straight. I still think of her a lot and, though I don't see her now, she still means a lot to me. I was very upset at the time and I cried all the time at home, although I'm not the crying type, more through injured pride, I think. By this time I had gotten married and had been living with Jeff for four years. Valerie used to find this difficult and so did I, but after Valerie and I split up I moved out of the bed I'd shared with Jeff and slept on my own.

I've had quite a few girlfriends but they all tend to fall in love with me and I don't fall in love with them as heavily. I don't think I've ever really loved anyone. I'm very selfish and I don't like things that get too routine. I've got a very busy social life with lots of sport and I've never really found anyone that's worth giving it up for. I'd been going out with a girl for eighteen months until I recently broke it off to go with a girl ten years my junior. I used to have lots of girls wanting to go out with me. Although this sounds big-headed it was true, especially round three years ago, but I'm usually unaware of it at the time until someone tells me. I find it all very embarrassing, although it does my ego the world of good. In the gay world I'm found quite attractive, but in the straight world I'm the butch girl who's shy and boring and, as I work with a girl all the men find attractive (I don't), they fall over her and she is very popular, it's not very easy for me. I occasionally get fed up with it, but not often. I find it very degrading to see her enjoying the men leering over her.

I can remember being quite shocked about my sister being gay. My twin sister is straight and, although she has had a fling with a girl, she is really into men, but she is very open-minded and does a lot to pacify my parents when they think I look like a boy because my hair's too short and so on. Soon Jeff and I are going to split up as he is moving in with another woman and I have to tell my parents.

FRANCES

In the first years of my sheltered life in Catholic middle-class Dublin I was completely unaware of homosexuality. No doubt I laughed at Dame Edna Everage or women with moustaches, but only because they broke gender stereotypes. I had no idea that there was more than one kind of sexuality.

At the age of ten, during a year in New York, I was astounded when a boy in my science class asked the teacher, 'Why do homos wear leather and chains?' and was given a calm answer about the role of clothes in group sexual identity. Back in Ireland, my peer group was not offered any sex education till the age of fifteen. I absorbed homophobia. I remember commenting that sodomy sounded disgusting and a friend reproaching me with 'different strokes for different folks'.

A few months after that incident I fell in love with a school-friend, Michelle. I told my diary that I seemed to be a 'platonic lesbian' (since my adoration was above merely carnal) but, no doubt, would grow out of it. After a year, when my feelings for

Michelle were even stronger and I was beginning to have erotic dreams about other friends, I admitted to myself that I was probably bisexual since, after all, there was no proof that I would not be attracted to men in the future. David Bowie and other pop stars were bisexual, so it must have some glamour. I found my position more heroic and poetic – 'the love that dares not speak its name' and so forth – than frightening. It was all right for geniuses to be a little abnormal, at least in youth.

My big break came at fifteen when I told my friend, Rachel, that I was bisexual. She said, 'Me too'. The relief was immense. Each being in love with a different girl in our class we formed a sort of alliance in coping-with-unrequited-sapphic-passion. Though I had a much more positive attitude to lesbianism than she did, I joined with her in assuming we would probably shift our attention to men when we grew up. She did, I didn't.

But for the first physical expression of my lesbianism I have to look back to the age of about eight when my turbulent relationship with my sister Evelyn (three years older) began to confuse both of us. I worshipped her. She spurned me by day, but was gentle by night. We played at boy–girl disco situations, nighties neatly between our knees. I was aghast when, kissing me, she put her tongue in my mouth, ostensibly to prepare me for boys. Once I recklessly told Evelyn I liked it when she put her leg between my legs and pushed. She went cold. I said, 'It's all right, isn't it, since we're sisters?' Evelyn never let me spend the night in her bed again, and we have barely been on speaking terms ever since. I felt ashamed of having put words on my pleasure and lost a sister.

At the age of sixteen my friendship with Michelle began, very gradually, to become sexual. We 'went out together' for three years, despite often feeling rather temporary and unmotivated about the relationship, since we were in love with other women. I discovered Michelle's body with rapture. For various reasons, it was a fairly one-way sexual relationship. Although we had to be furtive, and almost always fully clothed, in my parent's house, I felt no guilt about sex. Despite being a practising Catholic, I knew something that glorious and generous couldn't be wrong. So, although I didn't experience much arousal or anything like an orgasm till my next relationship, it was with Michelle that I first discovered joyful sexual expression. You can live through your hand . . .

At fourteen I had never knowingly met a gay man or a lesbian. I was completely isolated. An American friend of my father's that I met once was rumoured to be gay, but that was all. No family members, no friends or teachers – as far as I know. No role models nearer than Martina Navratilova. Convent schools are not as full of dykes as you might think! At parties, the more sophisticated girls in my class remarked that we all had a certain bisexual potential. We all flirted with each other, fondling each other's thighs under the desk or corresponding under pseudonyms such as 'the gay rake'. But I thought I was the only one for whom it wasn't a game. When we guessed 'who's the one-in-ten?' I dreaded that they knew.

In retrospect, I see a fairly clear division between the three or four in my class of thirty who had strong lesbian feelings and acted on them and the rest who felt a certain amount of sexual excitement in the convent school environment but never really fell for a woman.

I would have liked to tell my parents while I was still at school, but the risk was too great; though they wouldn't have thrown me out, it might have been unbearable to live with them if they had reacted badly. I was a 'good girl' and couldn't bear to jeopardize that. I thought they loved me, yes, but only because they didn't know who I really was.

My father found out by accident and deduction when I was twenty. He was rather upset that I'd been having a sexual relationship in the house, and anxious that I should keep coming to Mass and not get alienated from him and my mother, but other than that he insisted it was 'none of his business' and I was still his favourite daughter. As he got used to the idea, he became increasingly loving towards me, though I doubt he will ever talk much about it.

My mother I finally gathered the nerve to tell at twenty-one when I had left home. It turned out she had guessed and come to terms with it years before, but had not said anything because (a) it might only have been a phase, (b) it would have embarrassed us both to acknowledge that I was having a sexual relationship, something forbidden in the house to my straight siblings, and (c) it was up to me to tell her when I wanted to. She said all she knew about homosexuality was that a certain percentage just were that way. She thought it a pity that I wouldn't have children, but then neither did some of my unmarried siblings. It might be hard to be a trail-blazer, but I was good at that sort of thing. Above all, she loved me the way she always had.

Since then she has rung up all my family and announced that I am 'officially gay'. She is warm towards my lover, and so far has never tried to closet me in a family or public situation. For a woman who never knowingly spoke to a homosexual before, I think my mother is doing wonderfully!

MANDY

When I was about fourteen or fifteen years old my brother, who was eighteen, started going out with someone, but wouldn't introduce us or tell us anything about this person. So he was teased mercilessly until such time as he chose to come out. He told me by picking me up from school – in itself odd – and telling me straight. I didn't know what to make of it all, didn't ask anything or make much comment. Years later he told me that at this time when he most needed his family around him we all absorbed the news and scurried off privately to digest it, so he was quite alone. Eventually I just accepted it and realized he was still my brother and so on, but didn't think about it really, and certainly didn't think I could be a lesbian.

I wasn't aware of homosexuality until that time. One heard the word 'lezzie' at an all-girls' school but I never gave it any thought. Apparently, there was at least one other lesbian in my class and three lesbian teachers, but it was unknown to me! At twelve or thirteen, I had a crush on a girl a few years older than me, but that passed without incident. I suppose I didn't really think about lesbianism at all until I was in a lesbian relationship and that was after the not unusual reaction of 'I'm not a lesbian, I'm just in love with this one woman'.

With my elder brother involved with Gay Liberation I picked up philosophies of 'liberation for all' and certainly feminism. I would moan at the injustices that women put up with, but it was my brother who prompted me to do something. And a Christmas present at sixteen years old of two feminist books and a soldering iron was my initiation to feminism.

Gradually feminism and sexually relating to men began to appear to be in conflict, and a move at twenty-one from the 'trendy leftie' Avon town where we had lived to an honestly and blatantly sexist northern town highlighted the difficulty. Still I hadn't actually thought out the consequence, I just battled with my choice of men.

At twenty-three, as a mature student, I went to women's group meetings, totally unaware of the almost one hundred per cent lesbian attendance! But I became close friends with our student teacher, who also identified as feminist, and we attended events together. We were very drunk one night after a party and she, I and a male neighbour came back for a coffee and ended up in a three-way hug, which resulted in the man in a drunken heap on the floor, and she and I kissing. The rest I don't remember until the morning when I awoke to the awareness of someone in my bed and my first thought was, 'God, that's my teacher!'

That was the start of an initially happy relationship; difficult because of the extreme secrecy necessary, but we were madly in love for about six months. When it ended, messily and painfully, I had a short fling with a man, but I knew that never again could I have a sexual relationship with a man.

I came out to my family at various times, depending on the relationship with each sibling. One brother guessed almost immediately because I'm very open and demonstrative and I couldn't stop talking about this woman! My gay brother told me to think carefully as it was a difficult life to choose! But all have accepted it well and now there's no difference between any of us in the family and all partners are treated equally.

SHEILA

I had my first experience of a physical expression of my sexuality when I was nineteen. I was ecstatically happy. Any unhappiness I experienced was related to my family's disappointment, particularly my mother's, and 'hiding' my private life from family and employers. I felt a sense of shame in doing this and a growth of the loss of my general confidence in myself as a person of worth and ability. Over a period of six years these constraints affected my happiness in the relationship. I began to feel happy only when I developed the relationship in terms of sexual expression. Any strain that later developed regarding sexual expression grew from a sense of public disapproval of same-sex relationships – at least, that was how I interpreted it. The relationship itself wasn't the problem. The problem grew out of the way a same-sex relationship tended to be viewed by society at large.

My father was attracted to other men, but never had a relationship with one. I think the same may apply to my mother too, but she has never been as explicit with me as my father. I did not know of this when I was a child. My parents told me when I spoke to them about my sexuality. As an adult it helped a great deal to know that my father understood so completely and that I wasn't so 'different'. He accepted me as I am, just the person I am, including my sexuality. One older sister accepted me and wanted to understand. Mother was probably very disappointed, distressed and guilt-ridden. She tried to understand, but had a lot of difficulty in letting go of her dreams of my being married with kids and so on. It's taken us both a long time, but seventeen years later we both understand, accept and respect one another.

LIZ

I have a female doctor who is not aware that I am a lesbian. However, my father who is also gay informed the same doctor of his sexual orientation and received a rather negative response. She gave him two pieces of advice: (a) he should not tell anyone else – telling me (his apparently heterosexual daughter) had already been 'a mistake'; (b) he should *never* try to 'pick up' anyone.

My father had a nervous breakdown some years ago and still suffers from depression. He sees this primarily as a result of his guilty feelings about being gay. However, despite his disclosure of these views, neither his psychiatrist or the woman doctor mentioned above wanted to explore the connection between his failure to 'come to terms' with his sexuality and his 'mental illness'.

JOY

I was thirteen when I experienced my first serious lesbian attachment, but did not know that I was a lesbian, or the word. I attended a convent, and lots of the other girls also had relationships. We knew they had to be hidden from the nuns who made a great fuss if they saw two girls alone or talking intimately. I felt very strongly that my feelings were different to many of the others and in later years was proved right. We were told in assembly that certain 'unnatural passions' were sent by the devil, and that we must work hard, play lots of sports and pray to make a good marriage!

My first experience did not include sex, other than kissing and fondling, and I was over forty before I met another woman who had been a lesbian all her life and made love to me. It was the most amazing experience of my life. I felt for the first time that I understood what had been missing all my life. I had a sense of coming home and having my experience validated at last.

Because of my Catholic upbringing my early impressions of homosexuality were all negative, even though my father, for most of my adolescent years, had boyfriends, and many friends of both sexes whom I knew were gay. They were not openly so, but I realized they were all 'different' and that my mother strongly disapproved of most of them. From this I have developed a great distrust of untruthfulness and double standards.

I was eighteen and a half when I left school and was, at the time, very much in love with a girl of the same age. We never had sex but kissed, hugged, wrote each other passionate letters and poetry and shared a bed at each other's homes from time to time. She had several relationships with women and was trying hard to 'straighten herself out'. She began a relationship with a man at university and we then lost contact.

I married at the age of twenty after several other attachments, none of which were sexual, and none reciprocated. The man I married was four years older and an old family friend. I felt very drawn to him and went into a phase of thinking I could be 'cured' – though I realized immediately that the sexual side of marriage was a disaster to me. He knew from the initial date that I loved women and told me soon after we were married that he knew I'd leave him for a woman one day.

I had been married for twenty-two years when I met my first lover, and, although the experience was a real catharsis for me, resulting in my divorce, moving house and losing most of my friends and family, it was like a rebirth, beginning the life I knew I always wanted! Trying to disguise my sexuality for so many years had taken a great toll – I suffered two nervous breakdowns and various skin complaints for many years. The experience of coming out meant losing my ex-husband's family, my daughter (who has still not come to terms with it), my home and eventually my job. One of my biggest critics has been my mother, who is a very ardent Catholic. She finds the idea of my lesbianism 'disgusting' and we have no contact at present. It was apparent that my father still had boyfriends up to the year of his death at sixty-eight, but my mother refuses to discuss it and is now even trying to deny it. My brother and sister both experienced homosexual relationships in their early twenties but now, at forty-eight and fifty-two, are also heavily into denial. Both were initially support-ive of me, but as my sister lives with my mother I have no contact with her either. She does not appear to be 'anti' when we are alone, but with anyone else, or in public, she would prefer to ignore the subject or not be seen with me.

As a young woman, trying to be 'a good Catholic', I approached many priests and nuns. I was always told that my feelings were sinful and wrong and that I should pray harder, receive the sacraments more often and use the experience as a chance to become holier and closer to God! After my first nervous collapse at twenty-eight I was sent to a woman psychiatrist who behaved in a very primitive and disapproving manner. I was virtually told to behave myself, be thankful I had such a good, long-suffering husband, and get back to the kitchen before he changed his mind about me!

From then on, until the age of forty, I spent long periods in deep depression on tranquillizers, sleeping pills, bingeing or diet-ing according to my mood, so that my weight fluctuated between nine stone at my thinnest and thirteen stone at my most depressed. The only time I felt 'normal' was when I was 'allowed' to spend time with my brother and his wife who live in a large coastal town with a big gay population. I used to call into book-shops and clubs but never made a contact at the time. I just felt better knowing I was not alone and recognizing other gay people, knowing they recognized me. These things kept me reasonably sane, though it became harder and harder to go back to my marriage.

My earliest memory of reading about a gay person was *The Well of Loneliness* which I borrowed from a friend at college in my late twenties. I found it very sad, and didn't relate to a lot of the experiences described. I remember having a very heated argument with my husband about having 'such a book in the house' where my children might read it!

I am still constantly surprised when I meet someone new who has realized I am gay and finds it difficult. It is such a relief to be open and just myself at last – but it's no big deal to me and

I no longer ever intend to waste time on anyone who wants to 'put me straight' again. I have come to a very positive image of myself and of homosexuality through personal therapy and meditation. I feel politically that living openly as a gay woman is the only way to change attitudes and overcome prejudice.

3

Becoming

MORAG

My earliest recollections of *not* being heterosexual, at primary
school with my twin sister, half-heartedly joining in the childish
flirting games and rituals, meaningless to me but seemingly the
expected thing. Not myself taking part as such, merely being
there. One incident: a mock chase of a few of us girls by a few
boys, all the other girls a-twitter with excitement. I recall being
confused and annoyed that the point wasn't for us to run away,
but for us to be caught! This was achieved by the girls running
much slower than they were actually able to, in other words
females feigning physical inferiority to make males seem stronger,
more aggressive and effective. My sister's first boyfriend one
Christmas or birthday bought us both presents and I was so
clumsy I dropped mine, a bottle of perfume. I felt embarrassed,
both that he'd 'had to' buy me one too and then that I'd broken
and wasted it. It sort of underlined my gauche, unwanted, unsuitable presence in this boy and girl scenario! Another time, an
awful party at my sister's friends – totally out of it there too,
not into the whole giggly young girl scene, all dolled up, aping
grown-ups, dancing, posing, etc. I just wanted to disappear into
the next room and watch television, much more interesting for
me. An awful competition on dress jewellery – the girl's mum
had to be really sweet to me, allotting me some points to start
with to make up for my having no handbag or jewellery and so
on. I remember feeling grateful but annoyed at being judged with
the others for things I didn't bother with or know about. I felt
gauche, unattractive and out of place, but I don't think I really

longed to copy the other girls. I must have gained a reputation as Megan's difficult sister – oh dear!

I had my first boyfriend when I was about twelve or thirteen, I think, a chubby, bespectacled 'loser'/non-starter like myself, totally ignorant about sex. I suppose we held hands and kissed a bit, I don't remember. It was just social habit (probably my mum approved and encouraged in the background), no feelings of emotional, romantic or sexual need; quite sweet company; okay.

My first sexual 'response' was when my boyfriend's older sister's boyfriend kissed me. They were teasing us and probably offered to show me/us how to really kiss in a grown-up way. I sort of melted and can still conjure up the feeling. I swooned almost, and naturally closed my eyes to concentrate on the sensations. It seemed to last for ever and I was disorientated when it finished. He was much older and taller. I was vaguely aware of his stronger male body, very unlike my boyfriend's.

The first time 'homos' were ever mentioned (and I recall being avidly, genuinely interested, whereas my usual mode, in a world which seemed to offer me nothing, was pathetic apathy and a taste for escapism through books, scrapbooks of cuttings on films, theatre, and so on) was by my boyfriend when a fellow school 'friend' was mentioned. He said, 'Oh, him, he's just one of those homos', sneering. I thought I heard 'omos'. (There was Omo washing-powder in those days – whiter than white!) I had to ask him to explain and even then (and now) I didn't understand his definition – 'People who try to mould their own sex'. (Do *you* understand that?!) Anyhow, my overall impression was that to be this was dirty, sad and something to be ashamed of and *something males do*.

The 'homo' boy was treated condescendingly, like an outcast. I remember he would pester sexually, but rather for himself to be touched or petted than him pestering girls as was probably usual. I didn't get into all that until a year or two later. Basically, I just realized he behaved differently from the other lads.

I think I was always, from then on, tuned in to any possible references to homosexuality, though I didn't know that word then. I was confused as to why I felt a fascination for this secret knowledge. Partly being a 'loser' myself, I had strong feelings for the underdog, those condemned for some specific defect or for being or behaving differently. I didn't know anyone else who could share my love of books, words, poetry and so on. At some point, maybe that young, or at thirteen or fourteen, I must have watched all or some of *The Loudest Whisper*, the film of Lillian Hellman's *The Children's Hour*, about two schoolmistresses spied on and accused of being lovers. Such a secret subject (women, at last!) and such a discreet treatment. I must have only half understood, getting the atmosphere rather than specific facts. Also at that age I had a highly developed sense of justice. I probably watched the film of Harper Lee's *To Kill A Mockingbird* then too, or a little later, with a sense of passionate outrage at the suffering and injustice, seeing it all in strictly black and white terms, total good, total bad, no mature shades of grey. Anyhow, I never mentioned or discussed any of these feelings with anyone.

I was a rather serious-minded child, at odds with the flip easy way of my contemporaries, very introspective and passionate in my mid-teens about classical music – no interest then in pop music, hopeless at trying to dance, of course, though, with a friend of mine, I recall very studiously trying to learn 'The Shake' to some of her records.

My next recollection was seeing homosexuality mentioned quite openly and calmly in an essay that my brother, two years my senior, had written for his A-level course on *Othello*. He cited Iago's motives and Othello's confusions as stemming from their being homosexually attached to one another. I was really excited and amazed to find *that* dark subject as easily written about and by my own brother who, of course, 'knew everything'. Perhaps this also gave me a spur, a clue, to look for examples and references in literature and other books. If my brother could write such theories it must be quite openly discussed and written about; his teacher must know, everyone, except me, must know yet no one seemed to discuss it. But I still didn't know why I was so fascinated. Though thoughtful in manner I was not given to self-analysis at all. About this time, or a little later, I watched a television play called *Green Julia* with John Hurt and Michael Jayston – just two actors. The John Hurt character carried a photo of a girl (Green Julia) as a 'cover' because he was gay, but closeted. It was his alibi for not being with a girl. A sane treatment of a quality play.

We moved to a different county after my thirteenth birthday, so the following is all from that age onwards. I went from a mixed school to a single-sex one. There had been a fair amount of sexual petting in class in the mixed school (boys touching breasts and inside knickers), all very exciting and enjoyable. I was only anxious in case this was discovered by our teacher, but it was too much fun to stop doing it. There were also some flirtations (though I never expected to be fancied back) with one or two boys in particular. I was intrigued by their bodies and differences and I was tempted to look and touch when they teased me, but held back in case they went too far or hurt me. Also, however much girls messed about, you weren't supposed to 'give in'. I knew about penises and erections because of that gay boy having erections in class and begging me to touch him. Also, I must have seen my brothers once or twice at home.

I have very vague memories of a few girls chattering about having a crush on some member of staff. There were only two male teachers at the all-girls' school. These crushes were expressed quite openly as exciting fun but were not made over much of, sort of amusing but very forgiveable. I think it might have been the games mistress (classic!) but I couldn't see why they thought her attractive. I tried to imagine her appeal that way and wondered if it was because she was there fully clothed when we were changing before or after games, all at an age when we were very conscious of our bodies and undressing together. That's the only recollection, really, certainly no romantic attachments or actual sexual, physical lesbian feelings or relationships ever revealed themselves to me. I only once felt a bit gushy about the games mistress when she helped me out of the swimming baths. I'd gone under the water and was spluttering and panicking in a myopic heap! Her 'rescue' and firm grip on my wrist was stirring stuff, but it was her behaviour rather than she herself. I did fancy the headmistress a bit, responding to her a little as other girls might to an older 'father' figure. She was very dignified, rather masculine, but not butch, and cerebral in her manner. I admired her and felt she was on a higher plane. Again, her role and behaviour were attractive to me, rather than her looks or body. Her job as headmistress kept her cool and aloof, but I felt for her in her softer moments when her guard relaxed a little. I would have hated her disapproval. I wanted to be noticed by her. She was special. I admired her restrained manner, not superficial but deep.

Interestingly, at that school, there were two teachers who were a gay couple, rather typically butch and femme in outward appearance, as I realized later, but that actually made them quite believable. Role playing hetero parts perhaps made their relationship more real and understandable to me and the other girls who knew about them. I never felt this knowledge was negative. The general feeling was that this was just another piece of information. Obviously, it wasn't a bad thing if we all knew, for obviously, all the other teachers, especially the ones we liked and respected *and* the headmistress knew as well, and allowed and accepted it. Miss Markham and Miss Richardson were never snubbed by other staff members. On one occasion Miss Markham came into Miss Richardson's maths class with, presumably, a personal message. This hardly caused a stir though I remember being fascinated by their behaviour and interaction, how we knew and they knew but how it was never openly expressed or discussed. They lived together a few miles away from the school, passing me by in their car as I walked to school. Despite knowing about them and liking Miss Richardson for herself, a good-natured teacher with a good line in entertaining remarks who actually made maths understandable and enjoyable for me, and Miss Markham who taught art which I loved and thrived at second only to English literature, it wasn't a revelation perhaps because it was just there and calmly acknowledged. I was, however, much more emotionally and sexually tuned in to the English teacher who happened to be one of the male teachers. I was very concerned to impress him and to be noticed, not for looks or sex appeal as I still was, or felt myself to be an overweight lump of clumsy flesh, but to be recognized for any talent or intelligence I might have for English literature. A word of praise or comment or a look of approval from him really bucked me up and was important.

In my last year at school when, at last, the teachers began to treat us like young adults instead of imbecilic children, I formed my first real school friendship with a very gregarious, vivacious girl. I came out of my shell because she seemed so lovely and friendly and interesting to me that I just had to talk to her. I must have overcome my shyness and self-consciousness and become just easy and enthusiastic. I realized much later, with hindsight, that eventually I'd been in love with her. At the time, in all innocence, she was a soul mate in a lot of ways. At last I'd found someone to share my interests, especially art. At one point we both attended a particular art college enrolment day to see if we could get places there. My parents adored her like another daughter. We were always round at each other's houses.

I don't know what she thought of my gauche, ignorant ways but she never made me feel uncomfortable. Once of twice she went out with my brother but she was much too sparkly for him. We laughed a lot and she must have enjoyed my company and not been ashamed of me.

We kept in touch after school when she went into nursing. She had a steady boyfriend and, eventually, after qualifying, she got a flat on her own before they became engaged. The world of boyfriends and parties was still alien and uninteresting to me though she gave advice in an uncondescending way on make-up and so on. I suppose I was quite enraptured by her though I only felt this in a typical friend-to-friend way. I had no awareness of stronger feelings except a couple of times at her flat when her fiancé turned up. I felt that was another part of her world increasingly taking her away from me, but that was just change and growing-up. But I always felt a little self-conscious and ill at ease with the boyfriend. I suppose I felt jealous and helpless but was not aware of why! I put it down, if I thought of it at all, to my lack of social experience and my usual inadequacy in talking to or knowing how to behave with blokes. They didn't interest me, but I knew you were supposed to make a big deal about them and act in a certain way.

One occasion, however, is quite vivid when my sexual feelings for her and romantic feelings about her must have been growing and affecting my response to her. I stayed the night one weekend and quite vividly remember how special, cosy and warm it felt to share her double bed. We both read for a while before we slept. I recall how her movements under the sheets were disproportionately 'physical' and disturbing to me. Though it might just have been the unusual situation – I hadn't shared a double bed since when very young with my sister – but somehow her physical presence was intense for me, her perfume, though the feeling wasn't focused sexually or just on my genitals as such. I suppose I'd masturbated for ages by then, but this feeling was overall. I think I lay unnaturally still just to savour the sound and feel of her beside me. The only other time I slept in a double bed with a school-friend (and later on with my next good friend) it wasn't the same feeling. I was fond of her but not at all in the same way. That time it was just cosy and pleasant to be away from home and to natter in the dark before sleeping.

After school I attended technical college for a year and

attempted A-levels. I took shorthand and typing as I was a non-starter with regard to qualifications or career prospects. I got in with two or three oddballs. We used to chat and hang around together. The one male in our group I realize now was gay, very much a loner but with a strong sense of himself, who just didn't bother to join in with the other lads or girls. He chose and preferred our company. He felt no pressure from us. He only once made a reference to homosexuality but never even said the word. He talked about Gavin Maxwell, the author of *Ring of Bright Water* and observed that he was very 'strange'. Years later I discovered by chance that Maxwell was gay. This lad just said he understood how he felt and admired him.

The next gay reference was from the young English lecturer who was very like Murray Head, the bisexual in *Sunday Bloody Sunday*, in looks, when discussing Somerset Maugham, the author of *Of Human Bondage*, which we were studying. It mirrored in some ways the much earlier *Othello* revelations but this time in front of a whole class of very young and ignorant students. I recall a lot of sniggering, but the lecturer coolly stated his points and carried on. Afterwards, there was speculation as to whether the lecturer was gay (I bet the word used was 'queer') as he'd brought the subject up. He was quite tasty and wild-looking so I don't think the girls minded, but I sense the boys were nasty and belligerent. That was probably the first time I'd seriously thought of a well-known person who was known to be homosexual. I drank it all in and thought about it a lot. I was impressed that the lecturer hadn't introduced the subject in a negative way. It made me aware of being homosexual as a lifestyle, not merely in isolation as someone one has sex with, that it shaped a person's life and personality.

I had a bit more heterosexual experience, all experimentation, no real romance or sense of direction or purpose really involved. After that there were various jobs in a village a few miles away from home. I acquired another boyfriend, my first real lover. Around eighteen years old I 'lost my virginity' in a depressingly drunk and unpleasurable way. He had no finesse. I think he was a virgin too. It was all very boring but I liked having a boyfriend and went along with it all. Seems crazy now and a bit degrading.

Then I switched jobs and went to work in a small factory and became slowly infatuated with one of the women there. I was aware that I was lovesick for her. I tried all the time to be near

her and talk with her. I was so naive that I didn't at first realize
my workmates had picked up on this. I felt excited and alive,
really obsessed; with the sexual undertones it was good adolescent
stuff but maybe rather immature for a girl of eighteen going
nineteen! My true feelings dawned on me slowly and late. I
wasn't surprised.

I still didn't know how I could be defined as gay (or by any
word) but I never worried too much. I just enjoyed the sensations.
Although I was a bit tougher by then I still didn't enjoy being
teased and made fun of too much. My workmates just joked it
all along, never condemned or ignored me. Alongside this, my
hetero experience had awakened my sexual feelings and my
romantic and emotional feelings. I had another boyfriend, older,
wiser and much more fun and very considerate. With him lovemaking was just that, pleasant and comforting, though he never
aroused me.

At the factory, I had a weird sort of sexual interaction with
the supervisor. I was very aroused when she was close. There
was just an incredible air of sensuality about her. Very often we
contrived to touch, or make a mock caress. It was very sexual
but I recall no shame or self-consciousness. I don't know if she
was gay or bisexual; I didn't question that too much. I didn't
fancy her in a traditional sense; I wasn't in love. It was just horseplay and physical good fun, a real uncomplicated turn-on.

I never questioned why I felt like this about these two very
different women, never put it alongside the male lovers, compared or found it odd. I suppose, despite not knowing the words
and labels, I was calmly exploring and discovering my own
choices. I accepted that the guys were socially expected and
acceptable and part of one's status and the normal fabric of day-
to-day living. The other was real for me but slotted naturally
into a non-discussed, quieter, private underworld.

This all went on until I left home for a university city about
one week after my twentieth birthday. I went with a penfriend
who I'd got to know through a mutual interest in the theatre. I
remember an amazing double bill of *Women in Love* and *Midnight
Cowboy* at the university film theatre. Lots of homosexual revelations there. I was excited at the 'arty', worldly, joyful expression
of this subject. This guy I went with, Sudanese and quite unwest-
ern and old-fashioned about sex, was very embarrassed. I shushed

him quiet and sat totally enthralled. A grown-up subject treated calmly by most of the intellectually cool student audience.

Moving away from home and parents and the overall restraint and parochial world of home was a belated lifesaver for me. I felt free and alive, stimulated, relaxed and, at last, involved and part of life. I really blossomed. Initially, however, I got another boyfriend and lover, a white guy this time, very sweet and protective. While with him I became increasingly aware of fancying and being 'in love with' several attractive young women of my acquaintance. One young thing with whom I was infatuated realized that, but I just think she was cool and flattered, though not at all interested in me. I didn't feel too upset. I still didn't analyse my feelings or talk about them and I had never met a lesbian.

However, all came to a head finally when a beautiful, exciting girl started at the bookshop where I worked. We got on very well from the first and went about a lot together. It was she – asexual or, if anything, vaguely hetero – who guided me into the gay world. She could use the word 'homosexual' quite casually and easily, openly in a conversation. This was a real revelation.

Around this time, or a little before, I'd made a fool of myself with yet another infatuation, another colleague who also lived next door to where I had my bedsit. I was really gone on her and it was very sexual and physical. She realized and encouraged me in some ways, perhaps to see how far I'd go. I just longed to be with her, close to her, very excited near her. The worst (or the best?) occasion was very illuminating and the first time I was called 'lesbian'. I recognized it as dirty and an insult though, I think, even then, the word was strange and new to me.

We'd been listening to records and were lying side by side, fully clothed, on top of her double bed, me moving closer and closer till we touched, though neither of us said anything. I had an unwelcome date with my boyfriend, but longed to stay with her. I think she might have dared me to if I'd had more guts and been open about my feelings.

Gradually, my real falling-in-love with my friend and workmate and these other strong feelings led to trouble with my boyfriend. It was increasingly impossible for me to deny or suppress my feelings and needs. I never considered ignoring or fighting them, I just didn't want to be confused and laughed at. The guy had once had a gay sexual fling with some older guy and was at the time infatuated himself with Timothy Dalton as Heathcliff in the current version of *Wuthering Heights*, but he was ninety-nine per cent hetero, open and unashamed about it all. He even suggested an 'open marriage' as he didn't want to lose me altogether. I said, 'Sorry, no way, I've no inclination for blokes really and must follow this lesbian thing!' At that time, too, I was bowled over by the Nigel Nicholson biography of his parents, Harold Nicholson and Vita Sackville-West, and their open marriage. I identified a lot then with her and accepted her divided loyalties and needs, and admired her. I think, maybe around then too, I read Radclyffe Hall's *The Well of Loneliness*. I was very disappointed by it and a bit annoyed as the first-person's character was so male-oriented, not a real woman loving women.

I made a definitive end to my affair with my boyfriend, very decisive, but I couldn't go that way any longer. Adventure and a search for happiness were ahead of me!

My friendship with Sylvia was then a truly timely magic. She knew a lot of gay blokes and was in tune, though not herself gay, with the gay scene. She must have got me sussed from early on but led me slowly and let me talk and talk about my feelings. I expressed my 'love' for her. This was accepted in good part. She let me know she was fond of me, but could not return that kind of love, and that she had no bad feelings. She was the best, most supportive and helpful person to influence me at that very important time. After talking and being with her I could admit and accept my own homosexuality. I made decisions and found my own way. Thus I started the long-term process of becoming an active homosexual.

I went with Sylvia to my first ever gay club. Finally, I was seeing homosexuality as an almost insider. This was the start of learning and accepting my real identity from the inside, as it were, which changed my whole perspective.

NICOLE

No one ever told me that sex was enjoyable. I pictured it as a kind of fit that came on people every now and then, like dogs and cats in season. My mother emphasized that this was 'natural' and that there was nothing harmful or disgusting about it. She implied that when you grew up the desire to have sex would be irresistible, so that it was better to make sure you were never

alone with a man unless he was your husband! Not having sex,
it seemed, made you ill and frustrated. Since my mother was
very well read and I was sure she knew what she was talking
about, I imagined that all this would seem less bizarre when I
grew up. But it was a long time before I realized that sex was
pleasurable and connected anything I felt, physically or emotionally, with it. I thought it was going to be a mindless sort of
craving, like scratching an itch.

I can't remember anyone talking to me about homosexuality
when I was a child, though the children I grew up with used
words like 'queer' and 'homo' as all-purpose insults. I know that
I had heard of homosexuality by the time I was twelve, because
I remember having a conversation about Richard the Lionhearted
with a friend of mine. She told me that 'the same thing was
wrong with him that was wrong with Oscar Wilde'. About a
year later I read something about two men who went to bed
together, and that really surprised me since I didn't think people
of the same sex *could* go to bed – what would they do? I imagined
they must act out having sex by kissing and calling each other
'darling' and 'dearest'. I think, by then, I'd acquired the idea that
what was wrong with homosexuals was that they were always
pretending to be things, such as the other sex, since they didn't
have the sort of sexual feelings my mother described. Secretly, I
felt they sounded much more civilized than heterosexuals, but
somehow I got the idea that they were likely to be self-centred
and unhappy.

When I was about fourteen I started reading everything about
sexuality I could find. I was going with a boy who wanted to
be physical. He was clearly in the grip of The Urge, but it wasn't
happening to me. Most of what I read were marriage manuals,
one from my parents' bookcase that was probably the same one
that formed my mother's ideas, and none of it said anything to
change my basic (mis)conceptions about sex, though it did say
in cold print that homosexuals were immature, frustrated and
nice to know. Meanwhile I was passionately involved with the
friend who had told me about Oscar Wilde and wrote her fifty-
page letters. I told my mother that I loved this friend, and my
mother was quite horrified, not just surprised but speechless with
shock. So I never used that word again, either to my friend or
about her.

About the same time my boyfriend told me about a woman

neighbour of his who was a lesbian. When I asked him what he meant, he said she dressed mannishly, and when I asked if she really thought she was a man he refused to tell me any more. Looking back, I think this was the first lesbian I'd ever heard specifically mentioned and so the implications of my romances-from-afar with other girls at school and the amazon dreamworld I'd lived in since childhood became real to me for the first time.

When it struck me that lesbians might be like the brave heroines and beautiful-but-evil queens in my fantasies, I didn't mind the idea of being one at all; in fact, I rather doubted I could possibly be that lucky. This isn't like anyone's coming-out story I've ever heard. I suppose it just goes to show how much I lived in a world of my own. Or maybe it was a way of ignoring the practical problems I would have faced if I'd decided to live the way I wanted rather than the way everyone else did. I was sure that no university would admit lesbians and that they could be sacked if they found employment. This didn't turn out to be completely unrealistic since, later, my mother wanted to force me to leave university rather than let me live there with my lover. My father overruled her.

So, I just let things go on. Sooner or later, I thought, The Urge would have to appear, hopefully with some socially approved type of boy who could also be a good friend. I saw myself as serious-minded and sensible, 'waiting for real love' instead of rushing off into teenage romance in order to gain a passport to the social scene. My friend Emma, the one who had got the fifty-page letters, was a bad risk as a life partner – she was possessive, melancholy and critical – everything, in fact, the books said lesbians were likely to be. (She later turned out to be very heterosexual.) Another friend, Dawn, on whom I had a very strong crush for a year, never admitted to more than friendship. She was a realist; she said she wanted to marry a much older man who wouldn't bother her sexually. So there was no real prospect of a serious relationship with a woman, anyway, and I guessed I'd just been lucky to meet two women who weren't totally consumed by the urge to marry and settle down. There weren't likely, as I got older, to be any more. I felt rather out of things and expected I would change sooner or later. At the same time there was a sense of clinging desperately to the feelings I had then, even if they led nowhere.

When I was fifteen my family moved to another town and two

months later I met Kim and fell in love the first time we spoke. My feelings for her were so strong, emotionally and physically, that I couldn't ignore them or pretend they weren't serious. In public we'd learned to act the parts of intellectual, repressed, university-bound schoolgirls for so long that we didn't attract any unwelcome notice at school, but my mother sussed out the private character of our friendship which was everything a lesbian relationship was supposed to be: we were anti-authority, cynical and looked down on everything but each other, fantasy and books. We were going to become great novelists and world travellers. We also snogged a lot and sometimes wrestled, but that side of our relationship was never mentioned.

I didn't think we were the only ones in the world. I'd read about other women, and men, with our style of friendship, but I couldn't imagine a *group* of people like us. The whole point about us was that we were *anti*-social. I thought we might meet what we called 'interesting people' after we became great novelists, but I was privately convinced they would be worldly and competitive and not real friends. I was a cynic under my cynical pose.

It was only at university that I got a sense of the possibilities for *any* relationship. In some ways university was a very difficult environment, but escaping my family and suburbia made me realize that I had a chance to create my own life. I fell in love with my room-mate, while still corresponding with Kim as well as Emma. I read a friend's copy of Krafft-Ebbing and realized that I fitted his description of a lesbian so well that I might just be lucky enough to be one. But I had occasional sexual fantasies about men, and valued intellectual friendships with them, and I was still only seventeen, so. . . . All this seems a real waste of time to me now that I look back on it and realize that ninety per cent of my energy was spent on relationships with women, but I looked on being a lesbian as a qualification I had to achieve, not a description of feelings or a way of organizing my life.

At Christmas I went back to my parents' home and used every possible moment to see Kim, who made an offhand remark that suggested she thought 'we were lesbians'. I had always imagined I wouldn't like confronting a real lesbian relationship but, to my amazement, I was overjoyed. I ran all the way home that night and wrote a terrible poem about how we were going to have an affair. I mean that it was very inept poetry and completely sentimental, but my feelings were only happy. All the guilt and doubt I had felt about Kim seemed changed by the fact that she loved me in return. The next year she came to university with me and we did have an affair. She felt very guilty about it. I suppose the only reason *I* didn't was that I had spent so long turning the possibility over in my mind beforehand. I was, and still am, astonished by the way my feelings changed when I knew they were returned, and even more when we became lovers. I felt proud and very glad to be Kim's lover, and I no longer felt I had to apologize for the way I was so different from most people I knew. I could finally imagine growing up to be someone I recognized as myself.

SUSAN

During my last year at primary school I had one girl 'best friend'. We always played together and used to get teased about being 'lezzies'. I didn't know what the word meant, though I was aware that it was not complimentary. Two years later in my second year at comprehensive school I would laugh at jokes about 'homos' and 'lezzies' and knew what the word 'homosexuality' meant. I was learning homophobia by doing what was expected. Later, in the sixth form, I had very tender feelings towards another girl in the same year group. She was smaller and slighter than me, and I often wanted to put my arm around her in a protective way (not that she needed protecting!). I interpreted this desire to touch her as perhaps meaning that I was lesbian, since I was not physically demonstrative to my friends then as I am now.

An extract from a rare diary entry of that time (I was eighteen):

I don't think I can be homosexual, for Penny said she feels about me as I do about Hazel – wanting to put her arms round me. No, the thought of actually making love to Hazel or any other woman disgusts me. People are supposed to be prepared to accept homosexuality but I wonder how many of my friends and other people would feel completely at ease with me if they thought I was a lesbian. They joke about it – but the real thing? I feel very tenderly for Hazel yet don't want to turn her away from me.

I don't believe I'm homosexual. But I've never had a chance

to find out! No, I'm sure I'm not. What's wrong with being a lesbian or a 'queer', anyway? Nothing. But how many people would feel it was acceptable for two people of the same sex to behave like heterosexual lovers? Really, how many people would not feel uneasy or embarrassed? I wouldn't.

It is fascinating to read this again and see how ambivalent I was about the matter, and how scared, too, of being different from the majority in a very fundamental way.

When I left home, at eighteen and a half, I had never had a sexual experience with anyone. Soon I discovered the joys, or otherwise of hetero sex. During the next four years I had ten male sexual partners, including one committed relationship that lasted eighteen months. At the height of this relationship I envisaged marriage and children as likely, desirable and satisfactory, as did my partner. Since it broke up, nearly three years ago, I have not wanted to get married. I'm not sure whether I want children.

I do not remember, during these four years, questioning heterosexuality as the right way for me. I enjoyed sex with men. But, during this time, I became interested in the women's movement. This was rather tentative at first, as I was discouraged by my boyfriend's snide comments about feminists. When we separated I was very upset and deliberately became more involved in feminism as a means of support and of building up my confidence. I remember reading the chapter on sexuality in *Our Bodies Ourselves* and feeling my consciousness rising by the minute! I feel that my eventual ability not to be afraid to say I was a feminist was important later to accepting my lesbianism. For me, being lesbian (or, at first, accepting the possibility that I might be lesbian) developed from my raised feminist consciousness. I would not say that every feminist woman ought to be lesbian. Personally, however, I find it hard sometimes to separate the two!

I did not seriously question my sexuality again until a visit to Italy during the summer I graduated. I was travelling with an attractive and friendly American woman. I was very angry at the constant harassment we received from men, angry that they felt they had a right to accost us, frustrated at my feelings of helplessness about it. At one point I joked about how I would go and live in a feminist separatist environment when I returned home. Sometimes I think this was a very negative approach to being lesbian – anti-men rather than consciously pro-women – but it was a sufficiently extreme situation to act as a catalyst. If I had not had this experience, it could have been a lot longer before I came round to lesbianism.

Shortly after my return from Italy I stayed with a close woman friend. We talked about sexuality and the possibility that we might be gay. One night she was upset and crying in bed. As we were both in one double bed I cuddled her for comfort, stroked her hair and face, and felt very sexually aroused. She then turned over and went to sleep! A few months later she wrote to me asking whether I had wanted us to make love then; I replied that I had felt turned on, but unsure whether our friendship would have been spoiled if it had become sexual. She agreed with me on this last point. (She is now in a happy lesbian relationship.) By this time I was engaged in an ongoing debate about whether or not I was lesbian, and whether I could contemplate bisexuality. I didn't talk about it with anyone as it seemed too vague to put into words. Only on one occasion did I mention it to two close feminist friends, and even that was more an exercise in telling them where I was at, rather than because I was feeling desperately in need of talking about it. I wasn't upset or depressed about the confusion I felt regarding my sexuality. I was, however, uncertain whether to complete the postgraduate teaching course I had started. I don't know how significant it is that these two areas of doubt were simultaneous. In the end, I withdrew from the course shortly before the start of the third and final term, reversing a previous decision to continue so as not to disappoint my parents.

About a month later, I left that area to do voluntary work in a village further north. This meant living in a small community, sharing a house with people I worked with. I found this quite claustrophobic, especially as the village was in a mountainous district so I was geographically confined as well. Here I started writing my diary regularly – previously it had been very occasional. This was my only available emotional outlet as I did not know anyone well enough to feel comfortable talking about my renewed doubts regarding my sexuality and did not want to risk such a sensitive matter being a subject of gossip. My main difficulty was that Maureen, one of the women I saw every day, was openly gay. It seemed too easy to fall for the only lesbian available!

Then a woman friend of mine came to visit. We shared a bed,

discovered that we were both uncertain about being lesbian, and ended up making love! I enjoyed this experience, but it did not resolve any questions. The following passages from my diary at this time cover a period of about four months. I was then twenty-three.

> Two weeks after getting here and I feel so depressed! . . . renewed uncertainties about my sexuality. This is too small a place to have a crush on anyone, woman or man. Maureen said that most people come here to find themselves. That sounds too traumatic for me to want to deal with at the moment. There is no one I can talk to, or that I want to. I feel an affinity with Maureen, but she is part of the problem.

> I've had my first sexual experience with a woman . . . not an earth-shattering experience but, as she said, both of us are unsure about lesbianism as a way of life for ourselves . . . it has made me realize a little, for the first time, the oppression that goes with being gay – like being looked at for holding hands with a woman. Still attracted to Maureen, but not obsessed about it. . . . Is political lesbianism a serious consideration?

> Still as ambivalent as ever about sexuality. Sometimes I feel that intellectually I am lesbian – woman-oriented up to the point of making love. (And this despite having been with a woman!)

> The question of sexuality seems less problematic now – I feel that I am basically hetero, while liking to be close with woman friends and not entirely forsaking the possibility of a lesbian relationship. (I think this is known as copping out!)

Despite all this thought, I still imagined that I was sexually attracted to some of the men at work. I could not admit my lesbianism as I had nothing substantial to base it on. But a month before I was due to leave the village, Maureen and I became lovers after a long talk one evening. Before this, I had never felt entirely at ease with her.

> It's wonderful to be open to feelings and emotions. I feel very opened up, like a horse whose blinkers have been removed!

Catching a rare full-length view of myself in the mirror at the pub, I think – is this what a lesbian looks like?

That was last year. That lesbian relationship, my first, is still going strong. I feel very positive about being lesbian; I know it is right for me. As yet, I find it difficult to get this across to people on a day-to-day basis; I am afraid of possibly hostile or derisory reactions. I know that I have the right to choose my own lifestyle. I would not suggest to a heterosexual person that my way is more right than theirs, despite the fact that society in general would have me believe that heterosexual values are the only correct ones to live by.

DINA

I had a very involved penfriendship with a girl who lived in another Australian state. It was she who first raised the issue of bisexuality in letters when we were about sixteen. By the time we were seventeen or so, we were both able to declare that we were in love with each other (we had met when she came to my city for two weeks' holiday) but I didn't connect this with the idea of a sexual relationship. I was amazed when she told me she found certain female actors and singers attractive. During my school years all my adulation was reserved solidly for male stars. And although I had very little to do with boys (I attended an all-girls' school) I maintained the expectation that I would eventually have the sort of close relationship with one that I normally had with school-friends. I was aware of some erotic feelings towards my closest friend at school, but they didn't cause me any distress as my emotions were bound up in Philippa, my penfriend.

In the sixth form I remember that one of my friends who was head girl was asked by one of the nuns in confidence if there was much lesbianism among the girls. As she reported back to us she laughed and said she had wanted to say, 'No. Is there much lesbianism among the nuns, Sister?' We all thought this was very funny. There were jokes about convents, but I lived in such an emotionally repressed state when it came to my own homo-sexuality that I didn't give it very close attention. I remember when we were around fourteen or fifteen and one close friend had a big crush on the sports teacher. I felt quite contemptuous of her! I was quite anti-authoritarian and didn't approve of the idolization of teachers.

On our last night at school, a group of us went out and got very drunk together, I was in the toilets when one friend came in and started begging me to kiss her. I refused and suppressed the memory. Years later I found out that she and another girl had had a long affair at school.

During my first year at university I developed a couple of attractions to men, almost obsessive crushes, and yet whenever I was in a situation where something physical could have developed I pulled back. Meanwhile, Philippa had moved to my city and we spent nearly all our time together. She constantly raised the idea of us having a sexual relationship and I kept arguing that it would destroy our friendship which was of a very intense nature. Basically, I can see in retrospect I was really afraid of sex *per se*, and of intimacy that threatened to overwhelm me.

In my first weeks at university, Philippa and I went to a women's liberation meeting on campus at which a woman identified herself as a lesbian. This was the first lesbian I'd ever encountered. Over the next couple of months we got to know her and the women's household she lived in. But I think, in a way, those women had a delaying effect on my own coming out because they weren't particularly the sort of women with whom I would have become close friends in any circumstances, and they were quite into the mid-seventies fashion for wearing drab clothes and having what, to me, were very boring appearances. Overall, they presented me with a pretty negative image of what being a lesbian was. It seemed not to have much to do with me.

Meanwhile, Philippa and I formed a consciousness-raising group with two other women we met at a party, and before very long she and one of these women had a brief affair. I remember not being too upset when they told me, but on the first occasion after that that I stayed overnight on the sofa and they slept upstairs together, I could hardly talk to them the next morning. Still, it didn't seem to propel me towards Philippa, even though she maintained emotional pressure on me to have sex with her.

It was probably before she had the affair, but I do remember the first time Philippa and I shared a bed, a single bed in the house where she rented a room. We came in very late, probably put on pyjamas, and got into the bed. I lay on my side with her behind me, and she tentatively put her hand low down on my belly. The most exquisite adrenalin and sexual excitement ran through me, but I was so tense I lay rigid and said nothing. Eventually, we must have both fallen asleep.

Things continued in this vein for several months. Later that year we both joined a feminist collective which ran a women's centre, and got very involved in its activities. The collective was made up of around thirty women, and some of the most prominent members were lesbians. Even though I had by that time come across quite a few lesbians in women's meetings – this was the heyday of feminism and it was a big feature of my daily life – most of my friends up till then were like me, young women who weren't particularly involved with anyone. Suddenly, being exposed to the lives of women who I liked and admired, and who were older (in their early twenties compared with my nineteen years) and living lesbian lives, had a gradual impact on me. I could now see that it was possible for me to do this too. It was as though a blank page had been filled in.

A few months later, a crisis finally precipitated me into sexual expression with Philippa. Another woman, a fully fledged lesbian, asked her out on a date and they began an affair. I was plunged into a terrible crisis of panic and jealousy. I couldn't bear to think I might lose her. I still didn't consciously think that I wanted to have a sexual relationship with her myself (my repressions were still working hard). But the next time I saw her and stayed overnight, as I frequently did, we had sex. My life and my sense of myself changed almost instantaneously, because, in retrospect, the groundwork had been laid during the previous year. I embarked on a full relationship with Philippa and very soon was happy enough to describe myself as a lesbian, and have happily been so ever since.

HARRIET

I had my first sexual experience with a woman, well, a girl really, when I was seven or eight, but it had no name. I had just discovered masturbation and couldn't wait to tell Shelley, my best friend, all about it. She would often come and stay overnight at our house, so it seemed very natural that we would try it out in my bed. She and I had several such encounters. They were always great, but I never once thought about it in terms of sexuality. At the time I didn't really think about life-plans and so thoughts of the type of person I would spend my life with didn't occur to me.

I remember being told by my mother that there were a couple of 'queens' who came into the pub in which she worked. I remember her telling me that they were very nice and fun even if they were gay. It was all said in a slightly sneering way and the other adults presents joined in with the joke. I don't remember anyone mentioning lesbians and wasn't aware of meeting any until I left home and went to university at eighteen. Nevertheless, I knew about them and had come to the conclusion that I might well be one. In my teens I had a very close friend, Janet, who, like my earlier friend, Shelley, would often come to stay at my house. In the mornings we would nearly always masturbate together, but in separate beds. It was such a turn-on to watch her doing it and I suspect she felt the same at watching me. My feelings for Janet got stronger and I decided that I wanted to touch her rather than just watch.

I remember when it first occurred to me that I might be gay. I had a Saturday job in a shop and it was a quiet afternoon. I was standing day-dreaming, mainly about Janet, and out of the blue came the thought, 'Oh, perhaps I'm a lesbian.' It seemed like a perfectly fine thought and didn't seem too uncomfortable, but I was a bit confused by it. My problem was that I liked boys too. Now I was faced with the realization that I was attracted to both sexes and I hadn't heard anything about bisexuals. I went away on holiday with Janet and talked about my feelings and desire for her. It was all very good-natured, but she felt it wouldn't be fair to her boyfriend if we had sex. I don't think I was terribly disappointed, but it is hard to remember.

I then forgot about my lesbianism for a couple of years and had several boyfriends. It was only at university that I redis-covered my sexuality and that, strangely enough, was through a male lover. He and I talked about sexuality quite a lot and we both discovered that we had a bisexual streak. He was very supportive of me going along to lesbian meetings and encouraged me in getting to know lesbians and gay men. Unfortunately, it turned out that he got a great deal of pleasure out of being with a 'lesbian' and towards the end of our relationship was very insistent that I try to get several of my female friends into bed. We had an open relationship, although only in so far as I was allowed to go with women, but no men. He was very insistent that I was really a lesbian and he was the only male I could want. Looking back on the relationship I see how destructive it was in many ways, but it did allow me to come to terms with my attraction to women.

I have always had a very open attitude to sex, and homosexuality didn't feel any different to straight sex. It all felt good to me and I still feel that way. When I worked out that I was bisexual, it came as a bit of a relief and explained some of the things I had felt when younger. For example, I couldn't understand why I loved Tom Robinson's song 'Sing if you're glad to be gay'. Why had I played it so often and learnt all the words? I identified with it, but didn't see myself as gay.

The only problems around my sexuality came from my bisexuality. At university, during the first few years, I got quite involved with the feminist movement and, in particular, with lesbian separatists, which got so terribly complicated when I had a boyfriend. I had a lot of trouble coming to terms with the fact that I am attracted to men! I felt politically aligned to women and wanted my sexuality to reflect that, but then I would get the hots for some bloke and end up in bed with him. It is only in the last couple of years, and after living in another country, that I have made my peace with my attraction to men. I lived in Montreal, Canada, and there bisexuality seemed a more acceptable option. I am now filled with quite a lot of anger at the oppression that the lesbian and gay world, along with the straight world, has acted out on bisexuals.

I never felt that homosexuality was wrong or less valid than heterosexuality, even though I had no good role models. It turns out that I have a great-aunt who has lived with a woman for years, but I very rarely saw her and then never really made the connection. I didn't have any openly gay friends at school either. I just never thought about it in those terms. I knew I had feelings for girls and assumed they all had them too, but didn't feel it was something worth discussing. In fact, it amazes me that it all seemed so easy then. I was much more concerned with my schoolwork than whether I was queer or not! I don't remember any queers on television or in the media until I went to university. It now makes me angry to think how invisible we were.

At college, when I was about sixteen, there was a woman who kept following me around and buying me presents. I honestly didn't think about the way she treated me, I just assumed she liked me. It shocked me that I could be so naive when a few years later I bumped into her at a lesbian bar and realized that she had had a crush on me. Even though I had had those feelings about other women I wasn't able to recognize them when applied to me by a member of my own sex, yet I always knew when a boy fancied me. Without images of lesbians in books and the media, or indeed anywhere, I had not learned to expect and interpret the signals from women. How blind we were made.

My parents were very open about sex and always answered my questions honestly, but I never thought to ask them about alternatives to heterosexuality. I didn't tell my mother about being queer until I was about twenty-three. My lifestyle was so terribly complicated, with many lovers of both sexes, and for a long time I was living with a man, so it didn't seem worth getting into the maze of explanations. Once again I was confused about being bisexual and felt sure that my mother would not appreciate this outlook on life. When I did finally tell her she said she had known it all along but was very confused about my bisexuality. She demanded that I be one thing or the other, and still has problems with this and my non-monogamy. My mother's difficulty with my life is not so much with the sex of my partner, but more about the number of lovers I have and the promiscuous way in which I live.

When I told my sister, she said, 'So what?' and didn't want to talk about it any more. I was quite hurt by this. I think that to this day my sister believes I do these things to shock her! We have very different perceptions of life and can't really communicate about anything. I hope that things will improve as we get older. I suspect that she doesn't mind, provided that I keep it to the bedroom and don't ever touch my lover in public.

My perceptions of homosexuality have changed over the years. At first it was just about who you went to bed with and seemed to be as natural with girls as with boys. For a while I believed that I should only be with women and experienced a lot of guilt about the men I went with, but now I am delighted to be bisexual. It is no longer just about who I sleep with, though – it is much more political for me. I love the community I live in. I am proud to be identified as queer and demand to be treated with respect and dignity by all.

INGRID

I'm a radical lesbian feminist and I'm very proud of that fact, because it has taken a lot of work to get as far as I have. I knew about gay folk quite early on because I was taught at a music school by a very nice gay man with whom I am still good, if distant, friends. We all knew that he was different but we didn't have a name for why. I am also pretty sure that at least one of the teachers at the girls' grammar school I attended was a dyke. I had a lot of close relationships with the other girls at school, one in particular, who has also subsequently come out as a dyke, but there was never anything physical, at least, not then; interestingly enough, my first sexual experimentation at primary school, aged, I guess, about ten, was with another girl. We used to lie on each other on her bed and it felt good, but that was as far as it went. She's dead now, which feels awful as she would only have been in her late thirties.

I went off to university aged eighteen after having started on boys very early, as it seemed like everyone did that, and went on being het, but never feeling very satisfied emotionally or sexually. I didn't have an orgasm until I was in my twenties (omigod) and married for the first time, for the 'right' reasons. He was and is a nice man, but we fell apart because of family pressure and because he was going off to Ireland to do a job and I would have had to produce babies if I followed him there and didn't want to. I really had little idea that I might be a lesbian in those days, but had started reading feminist literature and questioning around that one. I remember reading all that lesbian feminist stuff in the seventies and thinking how wonderful to be one of those but not knowing how I could do anything about it.

Still convinced I was het, I went off to Europe to play music, got involved with another man, in Vienna, had a child with him and finally married him. Big mistake number two. When he broke my nose I left with my daughter. Husband number three (don't laugh – I did try hard, didn't I?) also surfaced in Vienna and I followed him to South Africa, where I was extremely miserable for a lot of reasons, although I had a good job in an orchestra, and eventually we came back to Scotland. He was so awful to me that I finally kicked him out and started a new life with my daughter, having made the decision that I would never relate to a man again, or indeed anyone of any sex, or so I thought.

Meanwhile, being back in Scotland had reintroduced me to a longstanding female friend with whom I had corresponded since university days. She, too, had had relationships with men but had subsequently come out as a lesbian with the help of the women's movement. She also has a daughter. In fact, I lived at her house when I first came back to Scotland. I had come back to London with my daughter, then left her with my mother for a term while I came up here and got settled into teaching, and while living at her house I was exposed to a lot of strong women, one of whom I really fell in love with, but she and I never did anything about it except becoming very good friends. In fact, I was quite freaked out at visiting her alone in case she seduced me! But there I was, around all these strong lesbian feminists, getting involved in the local women's newsletter and going to meetings and conferences and the like.

I attended a conference on bisexuality in Edinburgh a few years ago and began to have the most definite suspicions about where I was at, sexually. I think I thought I was bisexual for about two minutes. As a result of attending that conference, I started networking myself around organizations, joined Gemma and Kenric and eventually came out to my close circle of lesbian friends about two and a half years ago, aged thirty-five or there-abouts (omigod again, what a lot of wasted time and energy.)

My first real lesbian experience was with a woman I visited as a result of being in Gemma, but as she is a really difficult person it was a one-off. Actually, on mature reflection, it wasn't quite the first, as I did have the hots for another woman I met at a party years ago and we had a cuddle, but that was all. Then I went to a lesbian gathering in Edinburgh. By now I had quite a circle of friends who were dykes, but they all seemed to come in pairs or be unsuitable partners for one reason or another and I was getting desperate. I knew I needed to find someone to relate to and it seemed impossible. I can't stand the disco scene because I hate the loud music and there seemed no other possible way of meeting anyone. But it felt great to have acknowledged to myself that I was in the right place at last. And at the Edinburgh gathering I met the woman with whom I am now lovers and it is just great!

We are both survivors of abusive relationships, she with a

woman, myself with a man, and we really skirted the issue for ages, saying things like, 'One needs friends more than lovers', and so on, and then one day when we were visiting her my daughter, aged eight at the time, inquired of us when we were going to get it together! So we did and it has been getting better and better ever since, nine months now. I was a bit freaky about what lesbians did in bed at the outset, and very shy, but things are really good now. I feel I have come a million miles since all those years of getting it all wrong with men and am very positive about my lesbianism, even if it has opened up a whole new area of difficulty around coming out and to whom, particularly at work.

MARGARET

My family were very open about things like nudity, which was considered natural, but were pretty uptight and scared about sex of any description, and it felt like enough of a triumph over adversity for me to come out as an actively enthusiastic *heterosexual*, which I did. I have pretty much always been aware of feeling strongly attracted to women – my brother and I used to pore over the family's one 'art book' looking at the naked women, and I remember getting turned on, but that was as much by the suggestion of sexuality as by the bodies I was looking at. I had the usual sexual and emotional friendships with girls my own age between six and fourteen, then boys took over.

My best friend at secondary school and I were inseparable, and the boys called us 'lezzies', which I hotly denied without really knowing what they meant. She and I used to have sex on Sunday afternoons in her bedroom, though we pretended one of us was the latest dream boy, and we didn't call it having sex. I had a ready-made structure to fit these experiences into by then since my nice liberal parents had bought me a sex education book – *Sex and the Adolescent* by Maxine Davies, I seem to remember – which reassured anxious readers that most adolescents 'experiment' with their own sex and that this was a phase which I would pass! I remember feeling bereft and appalled when my friend finally let a boy go all the way – part of me was shocked that she could let a great hairy boy near her – but I was eager to catch up and soon did, rapidly progressing from brief fumbles with the local farmers' sons to a real relationship with a tortured poet two years younger than me – shock horror, that broke every school taboo! – and, finally, an enviable 'catch', a twenty-year-old young man from London (I was seventeen). We were both involved with the underground press movement and other political sixties scenes, smoked a lot of dope, hung out in the right cafes, toured a light show to poetry readings around the country and generally had a wild time. I discovered that I just *loved* sex, and we had wonderful, playful sex.

That set the pattern for the next eighteen years, during which I fucked loads of men, worked at egalitarian relationships with quite a few of them, and continued to 'fall in love' with women. This is strange – and I think it probably happens to many straight women – throughout my life there have been crushes on women, which I enjoyed and thought harmless, though they became more sexual and self-consciously flirtatious as my feminism made me increasingly aware that lesbians existed.

My first conscious recognition of homosexuality came in the sixties, watching a gay rights demonstration on television. I can't recall what it was about or when it was, only my feeling of horror. To me it was as if a group of lepers had stood up and proclaimed pride in their disease, so some negative messages must have been well and truly implanted by that time.

There are various significant fragments . . . my mother discussing something 'adult' with a friend of hers and referring to another woman's daughter who, they calmly agreed, was 'going through a lesbian phase'. I was intrigued. They didn't appear to be shocked. Now I know that my mother was only pretending to be accepting in order to appear liberal and tolerant. But quite suddenly, lesbianism became possible, though something which was hopelessly out of my range. For the next twelve or fifteen years I thought of lesbians as some kind of higher being, arty, cultured, bohemian, interesting, far far above my head. And carried on fucking men, quite happily, and falling in love with my women friends, quite innocently. I must stress that at no time did I believe, nor do I now, that I was 'really' a lesbian all along. I had a wonderful time being heterosexual, though it became more and more disillusioning as I became increasingly involved with feminism.

I didn't meet my first known gay man until I went to teacher training college and tried to get one into bed, and I didn't meet my first known lesbian until 1983, in a political group I was involved with. By this time I had had a very brief affair with a heterosexual actress. It was her first time too and she didn't like it much and left me instantly for a man who had just deserted his wife. But I had decided that I probably wanted to be a lesbian.

It was about two months after I decided to become a lesbian that I met and fell for the man I later married. We separated in 1987 and share parenting of our son fairly amicably. In retrospect this seems to have been my 'last fling' at heterosexuality. Then I met my first lesbian. I was fascinated and fell into such a state of helpless adoration that I would run from any room she entered in a panic. We are now good friends and laugh about my lovesick act, but at the time it was painful and confusing. I didn't talk to anybody, not because I was embarrassed or ashamed of my lesbian feelings, but because I was dreading that 'real' lesbians wouldn't take a married woman seriously. Of course, the community gives newly coming out women a pretty rough ride. I've seen it happen once since and I'm very glad I managed to avoid all that.

The next thing that happened was unfortunate, I had got to the stage of meeting lots of lesbians, hanging round in delight and fascination, and telling my husband that I was 'becoming' a lesbian myself. Then I read the infamous Leeds Radicalesbians pamphlet, and shrivelled inside. If lesbianism was like that, with all that vitriol and guilt and shit-throwing, I wasn't having anything to do with it. So I went to my GP, told her I didn't enjoy sex with my husband any more, and tried to get 'cured of frigidity' (yeuckk!), though I didn't once mention lesbianism since I have never really seen it as within the province of medicine at all. Very little is.

Luckily, I then got involved with a women's group absolutely crawling with dykes, fell madly in love with an extravagantly beautiful woman, got 'cured' of heterosexuality and we're still together four years later.

JUDITH

I clearly remember my mother telling me about 'odd' people. It was as if it was too awful to contemplate that it could not be spoken of properly and I was a shy type of child so I dare not ask. But then, what could I ask, as I didn't really know much about sexuality of any type until I was about sixteen. I used to feel like a late developer and I am sure I was one. This has been a significant aspect of discovering my true sexuality at forty years of age, after many years of feeling like the odd one out, but not knowing what I was looking for and often not recognizing what was there all the time.

When I first thought I might be truly different, as I saw it, I was in my mid-thirties. I spent most of my leisure time then with one particular man. We had had a sexual relationship for about five years prior to this but I found myself less interested in him sexually and he seemed to cool off me. It had seemed ideal in some ways as we had some shared interests and travelled around the world a lot together, but always went off in separate directions each weekend, me to my solitude and he to his elderly parents. I told myself it was ideal, but I knew it wasn't and I longed for a closeness he couldn't give me. I had some lesbian and gay men friends as I had worked as an AIDS volunteer. My 'manfriend' used to joke about me seeing my lesbos friends, as he called them. He worked in the fashion trade and said he was often assumed to be gay but claimed that my being around dispelled rumours. This made me feel angry and I'm not sure why. I was to become angry quite often after that. I suddenly felt very aware of all the anti-gay jokes that I had never laughed at anyway and, one particular day at work, I remember saying, in a loud voice, 'What's wrong with being gay?' to someone who was telling what seemed to me a very anti-gay story.

That was some sort of turning-point at work. People looked at me or just walked off. I have come to recognize that look, something between disgust and morbid curiosity. It is often still repeated but I get better at dealing with it or ignoring it as I try to do. I certainly don't bite like I used to any more.

About this time I became convinced I must be bisexual because I was getting very close to a girlfriend I had known for some time. She lived with a man but had had a relationship with a woman prior to him. I would do anything and, in retrospect, I must have looked a complete fool at times. The set-up was so absurd it could never have worked and yet I imagined it could. I was very lonely and just allowing myself to follow my inclinations. I was treading very carefully. I thought I would fit in with anything, a threesome even, so as to be near her.

Fortunately, my bisexual phase passed as an error of judgement for I decided that to be truly bisexual I should surely have sexual feelings towards men. As I had none of these feelings, I decided I must be a lesbian but felt unsure how to proceed towards finding someone. I remember driving into the local town one evening to read the number of Lesbian Line at the back of the toilet door in the library, but I still didn't know what I wanted to know! At that time I had many gay dreams about women I had known in my past. I found these very enjoyable and tried to get into a good dream each night. My fantasy world was much more satisfying than my real life then.

All this time I was just continuing as normal in my working life and yet my mind was racing ahead with plans. I eventually went to a few lesbian venues but felt unable to communicate my feelings to anyone there and just went home feeling miserable and confused. Maybe I was neither bisexual or lesbian, but what?

I eventually met my partner through a group I set up with the aforementioned friend. The objective was to discuss sexuality and labelling but we never really got off the ground. The group disbanded after four meetings but by that time I had taken an interest in Eva and hopefully she had in me. I then took what I thought to be one of the biggest risks of my entire life. I asked Eva to go with me to an amateur show for which I already had tickets. It was also the night of my forty-first birthday and I felt about eighteen and madly in love. Of course, she said yes and we have been together ever since as lovers and partners but still living in our separate houses. It sounds so cliché-ridden but I did feel on top of the world. People who had known me said I looked better than I had for ages. I felt I had come alive at last.

This was the happiest time I had ever known and still continues to be to this day. I felt like shouting from the rooftops what a wonderful thing we had between us and felt more sensitive than ever about anti-gay remarks at work. Yet, because it was so special, I felt more able to ignore the bigots around me. I even took the risk of telling my closest family. My two brothers were so accepting I wanted to jump for joy. Things changed when I went further and told an aunt, my late mother's sister and my oldest relative. She reacted with all the horror of it being a great family tragedy. She said she felt sorry for me, 'as if I were a mongrel' were her words, and that I needed treatment. She said awful cruel things about my partner without really knowing her and banned her from her house. She became obsessed about sex and what we did, quoting what she had read in the gutter-press about 'perverts' like us. It was a difficult time, to say the least, but I stuck with Eva, knowing it was right for both of us. My aunt never accepted us, but became a little less bitter in the end. She died earlier this year and I felt a sense of relief which I found hard to deal with. I will always regret not being able to let her appreciate how great my life is with Eva. Maybe I didn't explain it well enough, but anyone who really knew me could see how happy I was. She never knew me.

TANYA

My first experience of a physical expression of my lesbianism was at the age of twenty-one, in my second year at university. I had a very close emotional relationship with a woman in my first year and she had become very dependent on me, while I was going through a period of popularity with men. I had 'the upper hand' with her at this point. She had become obsessed with me and confessed to me one night that she was in love with me. I was, at this time, recovering from an unhappy relationship with a man. There were two occasions after a lot of drinking when she came to my room and we fumbled and groped about with each other. This was followed each time by me saying, 'Oh, my God, what am I doing?' and taking long baths the next morning.

I treated her very badly for that year. I would make her take the blame for what we did and I would assert my 'true' heterosexual feelings whenever I could. We only ever made love about six times. I only once stayed the night with her. The other times I escaped in horror. I would usually go to bed with her after she became upset over my flirting with men. In this way, I could make the excuse that I was only doing it out of pity for her and not out of desire. I was paranoid about anyone finding out and was embarrassed about being seen with her around college.

We were almost inseparable during the first two years we knew one another. Towards the end of this second year, my friend was becoming more positive about herself, her work and her relationships, and more attractive to me. When I came back from the summer holidays for my third year, I had decided that I loved her and that I wanted to make a go of it. It was too late. She had begun a relationship with my male teacher.

The next year was terrible and I felt rejected and isolated as a lesbian and very desperate. I didn't get over this relationship for another two years. I went abroad, after graduating, for a year, to a country where homosexuality is treated in an extremely negative way, but despite that I began to feel more positive about it and more ready to define myself as a lesbian. I even came out to some acquaintances there, which gave me a lot of strength. I only began to feel happy about it when I got to know more lesbians in London and began a long-term and very happy relationship with a woman who had been my best friend since I was sixteen. This was the most happy and fulfilling sexual and emotional relationship I have ever had.

JAN

As a child I was very tomboyish and a rather George-like figure (George, of the *Famous Five* books) desperately unhappy about being a woman. I began to lead a double life, spending the weekends wandering round record shops with a crew cut and leather jacket, assuming the identity of a boy. I was very convincing but was not aware of any sexual attraction towards women. However, on reflection, I do remember a fascination with female bodies which I vigorously suppressed due to my homophobia at that time. As I grew older I learned to fancy men and found that both relationships and sex with men were boring and difficult. However, I assumed that this was due to my inadequacies and I became quite depressed for many years.

I guess I should say something about how I became aware of my sexuality. I was going out with a man at the time and, as usual, it was a fairly awkward and unsatisfactory experience. One night I went to bed, having got really angry with him that evening. I had a dream that I was sitting in a women's centre talking to this beautiful woman from whom I was getting really warm, positive feelings. I didn't really interpret it as a sexual attraction at that point, although I guess maybe it was. Anyway, when I awoke, I knew that relationships with women were what I needed and wanted for my life.

My very first physical experience of my sexuality was being groped in passing by a woman in a gay pub and very nice it was too! My first 'proper' experience was with my first and most recent lover, a relationship which started four months ago and lasted six weeks. That was definitely a happy experience. As I said, I had assumed that sex was boring, full stop. It was a real revelation to me, how good sex could be and how aroused I could be and how wonderful another's body could be. However, I felt a bit anxious about letting myself go. I wasn't sure I could do the necessary or even know what it was. I got over this after going to bed with my lover a few times, although I still feel very inexperienced and rather anxious about the prospect of going to bed with a new lover.

I wish I had known about my sexuality earlier. I think it took so long because I was deprived of information as a child and didn't know a name for what I was experiencing. I think my Latin teacher, about whom there were always rumours circulating, and who is now a prominent activist on the lesbian and gay scene, might have been a good role model, had we not been kept so much in the dark. It makes me very sad to think that there are children out there who, because Section 28 forbids a teacher even to mention homosexuality, are going to be kept even more in the dark than I was. I feel as if I've only just made it into the light.

KATH

I first became aware that I was a lesbian when I was twenty-four, and at a women's college. In the first year I was there I felt attracted to certain women but didn't want to sleep with them, only kiss them and hug them. In the second year I fell in love with Jackie, but she was celibate, a 'political lesbian', and she didn't fancy me anyway. This was the first time I ever wanted sex with a woman but, of course, you don't always get what you want (especially not me!). So I pined away, and the object of my lust was sent to prison. On her release we tried to be just friends, but I found it very difficult so we drifted apart.

The first time I actually slept with a woman, I slept with two women at the same time! They were a lesbian couple at college and friends of mine. We joked about sleeping together for ages then, one night, we got really drunk and actually did it. One of the women, Sal, was very aggressive in bed, very 'butch'. She penetrated me hard with her fingers, which I didn't like. Babs, the other woman, was much slower and gentler and, in the end, we spent a lot of time together. I think Sal got jealous because afterwards she said she didn't want it to happen again.

The next time I slept with a woman it was Shireen, a friend of Sal's. She had just split up from a long-term relationship. We slept together the first night we met. I'd only known her for a couple of hours. We were very drunk and I had to keep getting up to throw up – not very romantic! She penetrated me and gave me oral sex, neither of which I liked. I wasn't physically or mentally attracted to her, and I don't think she was attracted to me either. We slept together because it was convenient. There are so few lesbians around that when you meet one your auto-matic response is to want to sleep with them. This one-night stand ended up lasting for two months. The second time we slept together I made sure I was sober so I could feel something. I also had my first orgasm. I got on top of her and rubbed myself up against her leg. I was so surprised when I came that I hit my head on the wall and nearly passed out! Once I found that I got turned on by rubbing and not penetration there was no stopping me. Shireen usually got on top of me and rubbed her leg in between mine. The next time I came the orgasm was so intense I burst into tears. And I didn't even love the woman! She wanted to penetrate me all the time, though, and didn't think it was proper sex without penetration.

Eventually we drifted apart. Sex without love gets boring after a while. She felt nervous about being an out lesbian. I think she was bisexual too. In the pub she'd tell me not to look at her, and in restaurants she was so nervous about people knowing we were gay. I didn't care, but she did. When we walked along the river once, I held her hand, and she felt very nervous about someone seeing us. I said I'd often seen women walking arm-in-arm, or holding hands, and people just assumed they were sisters or friends. Although, when I was thirteen, I was walking round the Boat Show at Earls Court and I had my arm linked with another woman. A couple of men saw us and said, 'Yuk, lesbi-ans'. They obviously foresaw my future destiny!

Eventually we agreed to part, (a) because I was going to univer-sity, (b) because she was moving and (c) perhaps more impor-tantly, the nature of the relationship. We pretended to be in love with each other, often saying 'I love you' when we both knew we didn't mean it. It was a relationship more of convenience than love. She'd just split up with her lover of five years and was still very upset about it. She'd often cry in front of me and talk about her ex-lover, saying she wanted her back. So I think she wanted me for company really, whereas I wanted sexual experience. So I put up with her behaviour which was quite bizarre sometimes. The sex was the only thing to keep us together, but that stopped being fun after a while. I was under a lot of stress as I didn't want to go to university and, in fact, dropped out a week after I arrived. I think this resulted in a decreased sex drive on my part. She was also putting pressure on me to let her penetrate me. I'd let her then hate it. We also disagreed on politics. I was a socialist feminist, and she didn't really care about politics. In fact, she could be quite right-wing and racist sometimes. She hated Pakistanis, even though she was half Pakistani herself, so we'd have arguments about that.

So, at the moment, I'm not in a relationship with anyone. I put an ad in *Spare Rib* and met a penfriend, but we had nothing in common and nothing to talk about. I've also slept with Sal. She's still in a relationship with Babs. They even got 'married'. But Sal stayed at college and Babs went to university. Sal had affairs and told Babs, but they seem to have got back together again. I just want to be friends with Sal, although sometimes I still feel attracted to her. I think we made love because she thought that was what I wanted. She tried to penetrate me, but I stopped her. I'm not really that attracted to her, and I'm certainly not in love with her. I don't know how Babs can put up with Sal's affairs. I don't think I could. But Sal is quite irresponsible and immature, and Babs seems to accept this. Sal is also very caring sometimes and very funny. She's like an opposite version of Jackie. Jackie and Sal both went to the same school and they look similar, short with black hair, but Jackie is very political, left-wing. Sal is quite right-wing. She is quite extrovert, where Jackie isn't. They both appear strong, but are really quite vulnerable. They're both quite 'masculine'.

I'd still like to try and make love to Jackie. We both had similar experiences as children. She was sexually abused by her dad, and I was given an internal examination by a police doctor after they accused me and my dad of incest, which wasn't true. This may account for the reason I don't like penetration because the police doctor penetrated me with his fingers. I felt like I'd been raped. Me and Jackie have both been in care and have both been in positions of powerlessness. I have a feeling she might not like penetration, but we haven't discussed it. I would like to show her that there is another way of making love. Sex is about power and control, and if I told Jackie she was in control and she had the power, she may be relaxed about letting me make love to her. The police doctor had total control over me. In sex I like to get on top occasionally, but I don't have the strength or the stamina! I'd like a relationship, but the right person hasn't come along. I always seem to fall for people who aren't in love with me.

SAMANTHA

I had an overprotected middle-class childhood until the age of eleven when my mother died suddenly. I had no brothers and sisters and my father found it difficult to cope. I was a 'good' child and didn't make things difficult for him. When I was twelve we moved to the city of his birth as his sisters lived there. I suppose he thought they could help him out, which they did. Shortly after we arrived we lived with his sister for a while until we could get a house. I remember that I had masturbated since about age seven by rubbing myself against pillows, but I started worrying, thinking I was going to die because of some damage I had done. This I now know was due to severe sexual repression as a young child. I remember being truly desperate and I honestly believed I would die. I solved this by asking my aunt in a round-about way and, to her everlasting credit, she told me that I would be okay.

When I was twelve I fell desperately in love with my female French teacher and this pattern of painful unrequited love or worship was to last ten hurtful years. I remember it coming upon me and I had to accept that something had happened to me. I felt very frightened and worried about it and tried to pass it off to myself as being because my mother had died. So I must have been negatively aware of homosexuality at that age. I told no one about my feelings and for me the next three years were spent in me being totally obsessed and infatuated with this woman. I can remember thinking and fantasizing about her constantly but not about having actual sex with her. My fantasies were often of something terrible happening to her and me coming to the rescue and making it better. By the time I got to about fifteen, I was so desperate I told my father a bit about it and I remember crying. He was okay and it helped a little. About this time she got pregnant and left and I remember feeling totally desperate and I thought I wouldn't be able to go on without her. I must say, though, that I don't mean I was suicidal. I have never felt truly suicidal. In the end I felt so bad I rang the Samaritans, who weren't much help at all. It was a man and he just said I would have to manage without her. I did, of course, and after a while fell in love with someone else.

I went out with a few boys from the age of about sixteen. I asked my father when I could go out with boys and he said, 'Sixteen', with no explanation of why. I didn't disobey, partly because I was brought up in a way that made me unable to cope with disapproval. I still have problems with this today. At school I pretended to the other girls that I fancied a male teacher. That did me a lot of harm because it left me confused and not sure of what I really felt at all, which was worse in some ways to just being simply in love with women. I used to go to discos with the other girls and let a boy pick me up so that the girls would see and think there was nothing wrong with me. I remember they always groped you and stuck their tongues right into your mouth and I felt very repulsed. When I was sixteen I asked a man to give me a lovebite and then I could show it off – pathetic! I always refused sex with men, however, partly because I didn't want it and partly because I was taught that women who just had sex with men were dirty or cheap.

When I was eighteen I went to a technical college in another town. I lived there during the week and came home at weekends. My father had died when I was eighteen and I now lived with an aunt, not necessarily the choice I might have made if I had my life over again. At this college I fell in love again, this time even more strongly than before, with a woman teacher. I feel it is important to note here that I have always, without exception, been attracted to women much older than myself. I was again crazy over this woman; I was desperate about her. I remember once seeing her in the town and following her around without her knowledge. I once sat next to her on a college outing and was so incredibly high just to be with her. It was spoilt by my thinking all the time that it would be over soon.

Afterwards, I felt terribly let-down and upset for about three days after. At this time I started going out with a man from the college, an Arab of about thirty. I went out with him for a year. I did it because he asked me and I didn't know how to say no. I also desperately wanted a boyfriend, however, for status, and also I wanted to prove to myself that there was nothing wrong with me. I eventually had sex with him because he kept asking me. I was worried about getting pregnant and went on the pill. I didn't enjoy the sex which took place about twelve to fifteen times. At the age of nineteen I couldn't stand it any more and, although it was very difficult, I finished with him. I then acknowledged to myself for the first time my true feelings for this woman. I remember masturbating and thinking about her and had my first incredible orgasm. I had another brief fling with a man a few weeks later, but I felt so angry about him pestering me that I finished with him. It was then I identified myself as gay.

Surprisingly, once having come to the decision, I found it easy and not very stressful identifying as gay. I was writing to the Samaritans. I eventually met this woman who was awful and talked a load of rubbish about nobody knowing what they are until they're twenty-five or so, and I should get out and meet friends of both sexes. I decided to leave it, as I was going away to do a degree. When I got there I had no trouble identifying myself as gay and started going out on the gay scene without worrying about it. I remember my father once saying that he hated 'queers' but that didn't bother me as he was now dead. However, I got a great urge to tell the aunt I lived with. I had previously written to my cousin who is ten years older than me and told her and she was fine about it. I told my aunt who, to her great credit, just said that it was my life and it wasn't her place to interfere. She has never judged me and is nice to my lover, although she doesn't really understand, or approve of my being gay. She has said that she wishes I were straight, but then only because I asked her directly.

While I was growing up and in my teens I didn't have any role models. I didn't know anyone else who was gay and it wasn't really discussed except for the odd remark here and there. I did have an overall negative awareness of gayness but that wasn't strong enough to cause me great problems when I came out. There was a gay teacher at school although he did not teach me, but I was aware of him being seen as a figure of fun and ridicule.

My first expression of gay love was terrible. I was twenty-one and had fallen in love yet again. This time it was with someone who was involved in a very violent relationship. They had met in prison. This was the first time I had been in love with a gay woman and she knew about it and encouraged me. Her partner, unfortunately, tried to get me to go to bed with her and I consented because I had to keep up the pretence of liking them both. It was horrible. I am extremely sexually repressed, although I didn't understand it then. When she tried to touch my clitoris, I couldn't stand it and cringed away, but she kept trying and said I'd got to learn to stand it. I was in despair and thought there was something wrong with me. I also thought I wasn't gay any more because I equated 'gay' with successful sex. Now I'd decided I was gay that was how I wanted to stay and, as I was sure I wasn't heterosexual, this meant that I was nothing at all. I later had sex with the woman I was in love with and this was marginally better. Eventually, it all came out and her partner attacked me and beat me up. I am a coward and no match for experienced fighters so I didn't try to fight back. She threatened me as well and I was terrified for ages and got quite paranoid that she'd come after me again. When I was twenty-three in 1983 I left the area and went back home and it faded away, although it has quite upset me to write about it and think about it again.

This horrendous story has a happy ending. In April 1984 I had the chance of a relationship with a woman thirteen years older than me; I took it and am now very happy. Although my sexual problems are not resolved I am happier than I've ever been since the age of eleven, or indeed ever dreamed possible!

Sex for me has always been a disaster area. When I was young, the message I received was that sex was bad, dirty and disgusting and this has affected me so badly that I have been unable to have a proper sex life. I still believe that sex is bad, dirty and disgusting, for a start. This may sound surprising, but it's true. I don't consciously believe this and I would never say it to another person, but that's how I feel inside; it stays with me and it's there at a deep level. I cannot bear to be touched on the vagina and cringe away involuntarily when touched. I have never allowed anyone to touch my clitoris directly, even myself. This I cannot help – even if I consciously wish it, I still cannot allow it. I have felt a terrible failure because of this, particularly in gay relationships. I could accept the failure with the man, but when I failed with women as well, it was a bit hard.

The picture is not entirely hopeless, I must say. I have had, and do have, orgasms. I can masturbate by rubbing myself against a pillow and I have had orgasms with my present lover; this is the first and only person this has happened with. I can do it if I keep my knickers on and she keeps her hand still. We don't really have oral sex. I find this repulsive.

My girlfriend has different problems. She has never had an orgasm with me or any of the men she has been with. She doesn't masturbate or get any pleasure from this. She was used to frequent sex and has enjoyed sex with me. She enjoys sex with me and has often got very frustrated, on occasions, because we have sex so infrequently. It was more frequent at the beginning, but now has dropped off and we go for weeks at a time without having sex. I've got to the stage where I don't care any more, it doesn't bother me. I've stopped feeling a failure and, as I feel my problems are so bad I'll never be able to overcome them, I just don't bother about them. My partner has adapted and doesn't bother so much now either.

MARIE

I became a Christian just after I realized I was gay, though for a year afterwards it never occurred to me that the two might conflict or that my feelings were 'wrong'. I only started to wonder after I read an incredibly anti-gay leaflet. I then started to discover that nearly all the Christians I knew, including priests and deaconesses, thought it was wrong to be gay. I don't want to give the impression that they were nasty about it, since they were sincere and caring people who truly helped me in a lot of ways and spent a lot of time with me, but for the next four years I became certain that I could not be a Christian and gay at the same time and tried to give up first one, then the other, but couldn't.

At one point, a female Christian psychiatrist was recommended to me and I saw her a couple of times, not really to 'cure' me, but more to help me be happier in myself. I really want to stress that, although I believe a lot of the counselling I received from my church and Christian friends was misguided, they were in no way 'ogres' who wanted to repress me or make me normal. However, their cumulative effect was to make me feel confused, unhappy and inadequate before God.

It wasn't until November 1985, when I had my first Christian girlfriend, that I began to feel a lot happier about it all, and to realize that a loving, committed lesbian relationship could be blessed by God, and that sex within these confines was acceptable to him. I hope you don't think I'm some kind of religious neurotic. I assure you, I'm quite sane! But it did take me a long time to dispense with doctrine that had practically been tattooed on my conscience. At the moment, I am with my second serious Christian girlfriend and I must say that my commitment to God is deeper than it's ever been, and my sex life more enjoyable!

MARJORIE

My mother confronted me about my sexuality four years ago. She had read my journal. I denied it. At the time I was bisexual. Then, two years ago, she challenged me again. I was forty-one and I owned up to my lesbianness. She is still working through it. She has given me a load of crap through letters about it:

It's not God's will.
What would the neighbours say?
Your brother thinks it's awful.
Your friends are poor housekeepers. (A terrible criticism.)
Where did I go wrong?
Don't you dare tell anyone in the village.

And the ultimate:

If you respect your father's memory don't say a word. (Or he'll roll over in his grave . . .)

4
Uniforms

BETH

I had feelings I couldn't explain when I was very young. I remember the first crush I had was on a girl called Norma, when I was twelve. I used to be ballboy for her when she played tennis. I used to sneak out of the dormitory at night to see her. We would just kiss and cuddle and we wrote notes to each other all the time. There were a few others after this before I left school. You were not considered normal at our school unless there was some girl or other you had a crush on. I did not know at this time what these feelings were but I know I missed school like mad and, although I loved my mother and father, could never wait to get back. My first experience was very sad. I did not get the same love back as I felt. I seem to remember mooning about all over the place and playing Tommy Steele's 'Singing the Blues'.

I was able to feel happy about the way I felt when I joined the army at seventeen. I thought I was home at last. I jumped into one affair after another from the very first week of my basic training. Then I went into Holding and Drafting while I waited for a posting and there I fell in love. She was called Celia. I was quite sorry to get posted to Catterick but there I had another love called Kit. All this time I had a girl with me from Wales called Ella (Spud). She always seemed there to pick me up when I met a crisis. It seemed fate that we were the only two who passed our exams and got posted together to Salisbury. I did make love to her. I took her to the seaside for a dirty weekend. She was always there though, looking back, I took advantage. And I saw other people as well. I loved Salisbury but eventually we got postings to Aldershot.

I hated it there, but there was a very large lesbian community and stacks of talent. We used to go down the West End at weekends to the Casino Club on Wardour Mews, and the Coffee Pot on Berwick Street, and the Alphabet Club. I knew a couple of strippers and we used to stay with them in Notting Hill. The army's own Special Investigation Bureau then discovered Spud and I and two other friends were lesbians and threw us out. At eight o'clock one night we were given a one-way travel warrant and two pounds ten shillings and sent on our way. While they were grilling us, which they did for hours, they recommended that all lesbians could be put right if they saw a psychiatrist. I told my parents that I came out of the army by going AWOL and working my ticket.

We immediately got jobs as telephonists with the GLC, all four of us together, and by sheer luck our supervisor and head telephonist were lesbians. By this time, Spud and I were having a fully fledged affair. After a year I met my husband. It was 'I understand you, and we can have a super marriage, you can go your own way'. I was the only child and I knew Mum and Dad were desperate for me to settle down. I said goodbye to Spud and married him. He was full of Irish banter. I can remember saying one year into our marriage, 'I will never change you for another man. If ever I left you, it will be for a woman'. I did want children and had three. I still adore them. I have never slept with another man and, indeed, eleven years after I married him, I left him for a woman, not without provocation though. It was only after he started playing the field that I actually left with her.

He knew all about her. We both worked in a hospital and she had to leave because people reported that we were in the toilets together. Well, of course, this was rubbish because we saw each other every night and didn't need to resort to this kind of thing. One of his friends rang my father and told him I was having an affair with a woman. Pauline is thirteen years younger than me. The children love her like their own. My eldest daughter accepts us. We moved to be near my parents. We took the kids and got a flat. My father, who is now bereaved, lives with us. We have bought a smallholding out in the country and my father has started a business for us and we are both directors. Pauline and I own the house jointly. My solicitor is just getting me a divorce and she says I will get custody of the children because my husband hasn't seen them for over five years.

TERRY

When I told a friend at work I was a lesbian, she looked at me with shock and disbelief and never spoke to me again. Another friend told me how courageous I was to come out and I was to be admired, but even she began to avoid me.

My mother told me one evening that she knew I had a problem but she needed me to tell her. I had been a bit down in the dumps the past few weeks. She almost fainted when I told her, she thought I was pregnant. My father took the news very badly and got very drunk. He burst into tears and said he wished I had murdered someone, it would be less difficult to come to terms with. That, to put it in a nutshell, was the contempt he felt for homosexuality.

Before I told my parents that I was a lesbian I had decided to join the army and train to be a nurse. I needed to leave home, and I wanted to be a nurse, and that seemed to be the ideal solution. I had my call-up date arranged when I came out to my parents. I was told that until I joined the army I must be at home by ten-thirty each evening. I could not have phone calls from female friends, and I should conduct my life as a heterosexual. If I did not join the army I would have to leave home for the sake of my two younger sisters. I would have to break contact with the entire family. However, if I were to try to overcome this 'awful obsession' I would receive a great deal of support and admiration from my parents.

At that time I had no homosexual friends. I felt very afraid. I was in a turmoil. And then I felt completely numb. I agreed to change, although I knew deep down that I couldn't. I had to find some way of meeting others like myself. I found a number in a magazine and plucked up all the nerve I could to ring it, having spent an hour walking from one telephone box to another. I started to go to meetings. I was young and painfully shy but I began to look forward to attending the support group. I also joined a gay dating agency. I met a woman, and for the first time in my life I was held and kissed. She was warm and kind and I felt safe and secure with her. We never had a sexual relationship. She could not cope with the fact that I was so young and inexperienced, but after ten years we are still firm friends.

My first sexual experience was two months after I joined the army. Emotionally, I was still very attached to the first woman

I had met. That probably explains why, sexually, the experience was a disaster. At that time I would have done anything and given up everything to be with the first woman who made me feel so wonderful just by simply kissing me and holding me close to her.

It wasn't until three years later when I left the army that I had my first real relationship. It had taken me that long to accept that a relationship was not possible with the woman I felt deeply for at the beginning. My parents became very fond of my lover and found it easier to accept my sexuality. My mother said a prayer that I would change. I threw a coin into a wishing well, hoping that my parents would change. I seem to have won!

JEAN

My background was somewhat sheltered and protected, being the only daughter of a Methodist minister. It was not until I began my nursing training at age eighteen that I became aware that it was possible for two men to have a sexual relationship, and not until sometime later than that did I realize what my own feelings were about. The way I discovered about gay men was that two men were admitted to the men's ward on which I was working. Great effort was made to ensure they were at opposite ends of a very long ward and staff were instructed to ensure that at no time did these men go to the loo at the same time. Being my naturally curious self, I dared to ask 'Why?', only to be given the somewhat oblique answer that men like that had 'unclean habits and would give each other VD and that their friendship was perverted'. This was in 1973!

LISA

When I started nursing I found myself increasingly drawn to women, but pushed it to the back of my mind as unacceptable. I had no knowledge of any of my friends or relations being homosexual, and it never occurred to me to ring a helpline and get some advice. I did actually confide in a friend but, although she was very good, she didn't really know how to help me.

I persevered with men and actually managed to have two (for me) long-term relationships. I never felt quite at ease, though. I was, by this time, in the army and it was there that I fell in love

with one of my friends. It caused me to re-examine the feelings
I had suppressed for so long, and I finally came to terms with
the fact that I was more attracted to women than men. I was
very depressed for a while – the army is not exactly the most
friendly environment for homosexuals. It has some disgustingly
antiquated practices such as the Special Investigations Branch,
which has the right to search your room, read personal letters,
etc. if they suspect you of harbouring 'deviant' tendencies. I came
out of the army and returned to my old hospital.

TINA

I come from a northern fishing town which sports the same
provincial attitudes it did when I was growing up. My family
moved here from a multiracial city in Wales in the late 1950s,
and I was born here in the early sixties. The number of other
black or mixed-race families living here at the time didn't make
double figures, and there was no black community of any description. We were subjected to a great deal of prejudice, verbal and
sometimes physical abuse, and, as our extended family lived
nearly three hundred miles away, we had no support network at
all. Presumably, the other black families living here suffered the
same fate. None of us ever communicated. It must have been a
huge shock for my family who had previously lived in a city
where they had been supported by their own community, but
for me the hostility was a way of life. My childhood was spent
feeling very isolated, and I guess the issue of my sexuality took
a back seat to the problems created by my more visible 'difference'. People seemed to react very badly towards black people,
lesbians and gay men, in fact anyone they perceived to be different
in some way; the images I got then of homosexuality and race
were very negative and, although things have improved since my
childhood, the general atmosphere here is still quite uncomfortable.

I joined the army before my eighteenth birthday and moved
down to the south of England to do my training, and it was then
that I saw other women who thought the same way as I did and
with whom I could identify. The feeling I had when I walked
into the NAAFI for the first time and saw this group of strong,
confident and happy women who bought me a drink and immediately took me under their wing is indescribable. Suffice it to say

that I felt completely at home in company for the first time in my life, and there was a kind of mutual, unspoken understanding that I had never experienced before. No one spoke about lesbianism at all, but they recognized me and I recognized them. More importantly for me, I suddenly recognized myself, and I'm very relieved that the revelation came under such positive circumstances. My lesbianism wasn't something I felt I had to come to terms with; that experience purely provided me with a name for my feelings, and it was something that made me very relieved and happy.

I phoned my mother one night soon afterwards and told her I was a lesbian as part of our general conversation. I told her more for her information than to 'confess', and I think she accepted it as such. I think she discussed it with my family, but no one ever questioned my decision.

My lover and I have been together for almost two years. We met at a dance in her home town one night, introduced by a woman acquaintance. Where she comes from most relationships begin from meeting in a disco; there are quite a few nightclubs which cater for lesbians and gay men, and consequently they are the main meeting places. Where we live now, in my home town, there are very few social activities. Women tend not to congregate in large numbers here. There are lots of small cells of lesbians, quite separate from one another, and it is fairly difficult to flit from one to another. Who one meets is largely dependent upon which cell one belongs to, which is quite restrictive.

Our lovership is constantly adjusting – there is always a need for compromise within a relationship. We both of us recognize that we are individuals with our own outlook on life, but that in order for a joint agreement like a relationship to work we have to modify certain attitudes and maybe give up certain things we enjoy doing alone that might place a strain on us as a couple. For instance, before I met my present lover, I had a number of friends with whom I had a 'flirting' relationship, which meant that we could have progressed to a sexual relationship at any time but for the moment were enjoying the 'play', the flirt. I found this activity particularly fascinating because it was something I had never experienced before. I enjoyed being free (out of a relationship) and making my own choices about whether or not I slept with someone, without having to consider a lover. I have always been in a long-term relationship and have never been free to have other lovers, so this was a new experience. When I met my present lover, I gave up my group of friends because I couldn't relate to them on the same level any more; it caused friction in my relationship. It makes me sad, but I also understand that if the situation had been reversed, and it was my lover who had been relating to other women in this way, then I'd have felt threatened too.

When things are going well between us, when we feel really close, then sex isn't really very important. When we're arguing, or feel vulnerable, sex then springs to the top of the list of 'things wrong with our relationship'. Suddenly, one of us feels we're no longer sexually attractive to the other, irrespective of how often we're having sex or how good it is. Normally, neither of us is particularly highly sexed. We make love about once a week, if we remember! But we're both very tactile and enjoy loving each other without necessarily going the whole way. Occasionally, we experiment, doing stuff one of us thinks the other might enjoy, but on the whole I think we both of us revel in being physically close, holding each other, stroking each other's body.

My lover hasn't come out to her family, so she feels under a lot of pressure to conform. She's in her thirties and her parents feel she should be married by now. Consequently, she often feels torn between what she feels she should be doing and living her life the way that makes her happy. By contrast, I've been out since I was eighteen, so my family has no illusions. However, they have often interfered in my lesbian relationships and have created friction and ill-feeling where there was no call for any, so I have largely excluded them from my life. I have only occasional contact with my mother and my oldest sister, and keep them both at arm's length. It's sad, but it's the only way I can be free to live my own life.

Apart from our families, we don't have much outside pressure – the occasional insult from some idiot in the street, but not much more than that. We feel like an ordinary couple and we act as such. We know that we're discriminated against and that lots of people have a problem with our sexuality, but that's their problem and I think we would only take on board situations that directly affect our living situation, such as problems with our landlord or the DHSS. Fortunately, we haven't had any difficulties in this respect yet. On the street, I've had one or two confrontations with straight men who have felt threatened by my sexuality, but it's turned out okay.

When I was much younger, I often wished that I could marry the lover I was with. It was a fairy-tale thing, a happily-ever-after seal on a relationship. Now I realize that, if such a marriage was legal in this country, I would be very reluctant to take the step unless I was absolutely sure that the relationship was completely stable. I think there should be an option like this for lesbian and gay couples, both as a declaration of love and as legal security for a partner who is left when a lover dies, or couples splitting up. But I also think that, for many of us, there would be difficulties with taking such a contract seriously because of the casual nature of our social environment. I think that often we don't take ourselves seriously as people with a different, but equally valid, sexual and political identity, so maybe we'd have to re-educate ourselves quite extensively in order to accept something as formal as marriage into our collection of life choices.

5

Out

LOUISE

I am definitely out. I have reached the stage where I see no point
in hiding my sexuality to most people with whom I have anything
more than casual contact. Besides which, I have a feeling that I
look like and dress like and act like such a lesbian that if people
don't get the hint then it's obviously something so far outside
their scope of life that it would be unkind to spell things out in
words of one syllable.

I don't recall coming out as a grand event. It wasn't like I was
the only person who knew, followed by an announcement in all
the national newspapers. It was more gradual than that. I told
my best friend at school that I was in love with one of the
teachers, which was fine because this friend had a crush on one
of the other girls at the time. So we shared crushes for a while.
I told a few friends after I'd left school and they all had roughly
the same reaction, that I was still their friend, which was nice
(and a good thing too. I told one friend as we sat in a bandstand
in Ballarat in South Australia. If she'd taken it badly the following
three months touring Australia would have been tense, to say the
least!)

The first member of my family I came out to was my sister,
when I was unceremoniously dumped by the woman I'd thought
was going to be 'It' for my whole life. I was totally hysterical at
the time, so my sister hardly had the chance to react badly, she
was too shocked to make any judgements. My mother already
knew by the time I got round to telling her because one of her
workmates had got me sussed and told her and calmed her down
and explained everything. So it was no big news to her, and she

was okay about it. I didn't tell my father for ages and, when I eventually did, it was a great relief to him. I had been trekking across town twice a week to go to a pub when there's one just round the corner, and he'd been wondering why I bothered. He'd gradually decided that I was working as a barmaid in some sleazy joint and that was why I was so secretive. When I told him it was a women's bar and I went there because I'm a lesbian, he said, 'Oh, that's a relief then'! My parents, by the way, are dead sound and completely wonderful and supportive and, looking back, I wonder why I left it so long. But you can't be sure, can you? And I didn't want to hurt them.

I came out at college by having a large poster of two women locked in an embrace on my wall. It worked a treat. To start with, I had come out to individuals but no one was too freaked out, especially as I had a girlfriend, so they weren't worried I was going to pounce.

Because I've never had a severely negative reaction to my face, I've not held back on coming out since I started college. It's not so much 'coming out' as just being me, and part of being me is that I'm a dyke, take it or leave it. I've always been out at work. I've never said clearly, 'By the way, I'm a lesbian', but I just let it be known. I talk about my partner or girlfriend and if people are too horrified they'll steer clear of me the next time. But then I work in a nice intellectual atmosphere where most of my colleagues read *The Guardian* and it would be most improper of them to react otherwise. I think some of them actually think it gives them credibility to have a lesbian couple as friends. But I am fully aware that a large section of the population would happily beat me up and/or rape me if the situation permitted it. So I subscribe to the ostrich school of life and avoid these people and those situations as much as possible. I would never make it clear that I was a dyke if I thought there was any physical danger. I'm not a martyr to the cause.

Only once did I make an outrageous and gratuitous reference to my sexuality and now I feel quite guilty about it, but it was such fun at the time. I was in the ladies' loo at a service station and got stared at by Mrs Het, who coldly informed me that this was the ladies. I get that quite a lot and usually just agree with them that, indeed, it *is* the ladies and let them figure it out. But that time (and God knows what possessed me to say it!) I said, 'What's the matter? Don't you know a lesbian when you see one?'

She was suitably taken aback and shot into the nearest cubicle and bolted the door. . . .

ANDREA

You suggest that coming out is a public affirmation or celebration of one's sexuality. Oh, dear me, no. A fight. To be me. To be recognized as me. To avoid being lynched for being me. To knock some goddamn sense into the world.

My first coming out was to myself, when the penny finally dropped that *that* was what I was. So, that's what I am – a lesbian. Just to say that out loud still scares me. And amazes me. No, the sky doesn't fall just because I say I'm a lesbian. But someday it will, I'm convinced of it. Sometime I'll say it to the wrong person in the wrong place and lose my job, my flat, my career and my family in one fell swoop, I know it.

So, I say it to the people I work with, again and again, because they'd love to forget or pretend that, after all, if they keep quiet long enough maybe I'll end up like them. And every time there's a shock in the air. Their faces twitch slightly, the kind of contortion that says, 'I'm telling myself not to react. After all, it's the eighties and I'm a right-on leftie feminist, but why does she have to keep reminding me she's queer?' And then they get all reasonable and lecture *me* on equal rights. Jesus, sometimes I'd love to just walk right out of there.

But no, I NEVER, NEVER tell my pupils, their parents, the cleaners, the schoolkeeper, my assistant, my landlady or my parents. Why court disaster? Well, yes, I know why. Believe me, I feel the full force of Harvey Milk's impassioned plea for courage. But I'm a coward. I would love nothing better than to believe that if I told the whole world, the world would mildly turn round, pat me on the head and say, 'Yes, dear, we understand'. But the world happens to be a nasty, vicious place where people love nothing better than a touch of violence to spice up their lives and I'm more interested in survival than heroics.

My God, I'm getting reactionary in my old age. You wouldn't believe this is the same person who, shivering with terror, used to walk around wearing a lesbian badge on my jacket lapel and who still drags herself kicking and screaming on to both the Lesbian Strength and Gay Pride marches every year, who founded a primary teachers' lesbian and gay group in a *teachers' centre*, for heaven's sake, and attends various lesbian and gay group meetings around the city. . . .

So what is this kamikaze tendency to scream things from the rooftops and then duck behind the balustrade for fear of imaginary missiles? Advantages? One small space I can call mine. At work, at home, in bits of the world I can be myself. But even there, straight people don't really understand.

I was listening to Radio 4 one day, to a marvellous gay man whom I admire enormously for his incredible courage. He was talking about 'the intolerable strain of living in two worlds' and the need for us to 'reconcile' these two worlds. Well, that's it. He wasn't talking about coming out, but it hits the nail on the head, nevertheless. Coming out is my way of bringing the two halves of my world together so that I can stay sane. If I don't try, they'll go spinning off in opposite directions, tearing me apart as they do so.

ROSEMARY

The advantages in coming out are the sense of personal freedom, the loss of fear. It means a lot to me when I hear even a mildly anti-gay remark, for example, 'All this public spending on lesbians and gays', to say, 'Look, I'm gay and that's not the truth'. More so since AIDS. I feel my arguments have more weight when talking, say, to a minibus driver who seemed to think he could get AIDS from hotel linen. I could say, 'I'm gay, and you don't get AIDS like that'. This resulted in a rather comic conversation with me yelling advice on condoms from the back of the bus. He'd seriously been talking of cancelling his holiday 'because of all these gays about'. He's since driven me without any nonsense, except racist nonsense, which seems a bit harder to eradicate.

I feel too it's important for me to be identified as a lesbian for the sake of people who are still in the closet. Even if they never come out it must be some source of solidarity to know there are people who are out. I remember when I was still in the closet the joy of seeing other lesbians on television; there they were, real people like me, my own people visible for once. And it's wonderful feeling part of the lesbian and gay community, being recognized and recognizing others, being part of this 'out' network. Maybe this is even better than being part of an accepting, largely het family? It would, of course, be nice to have both! But I think that because of this connection with other lesbians and gays I don't miss family support.

Apart from them and my doctor who is, I think, Catholic, and who I don't know at all as I see him as little as possible, I don't think I do select now who I come out to. It just seems to happen. For instance, when one het woman I met at a community centre was telling me about her courtship, and added, 'I'll find a nice man for you'. I said 'I don't want one, I'm a lesbian' and she simply rejoined, 'Oh, I'm quite the other way'.

Once a minicab driver was telling me, on a long journey, about the sort of work he had and how he regularly picked up artistes from gay pubs, and I said something like, 'Yes, there are a lot of good venues around here'. He said 'How do you know?' and I said, 'I'm a lesbian'. He went very pale and it seemed clear to me he was a closet gay because, although he said 'I'm not married, but I'm not gay', he went on talking about it and then said, 'But it's wrong to be gay, isn't it?' I said, no, it wasn't, gays could act responsibly to each other and have good relationships and no love was wrong if it wasn't exploitative. I don't know if I was right about him and if it helped him at all, but if I'd been in the closet perhaps we wouldn't have had the conversation at all. As he was a local cabby, I think maybe he'd heard I was gay but hadn't expected me to say so.

I'm not religious so I can't say anything about telling priests. One could, I suppose, always ring them up anonymously and sound them out on their attitudes to gays beforehand. One rather closeted woman I knew, who came out to her priest, found him not anti-gay. He just said 'Do the best you can'.

I think I would not come out to medical people deliberately. If they learn about me from other sources then that is different. I think they are poorly educated or trained as far as sexuality is concerned. I know a woman who had 'homosexual' scrawled in her medical file. While I realize this could be beneficial if you need to establish your lover as next of kin, I feel uneasy about it. I don't think medical files are confidential. I suppose I don't want that fact about me in bold print in a hospital when I am helpless and at the mercy of medics there. I've spent too much time in hospitals to have any illusions about still having much control over my life in there and the sort of treatment I'd get. And nuns and religious maniacs tend to loom up in hospital. I once had to endure a nun going on and on about my loss of religion which she'd tracked down in my file. Imagine having to depend on bedpans from someone who chooses to go on and on about gays.

REBECCA

I had my first lesbian relationship at university. It was a very agonizing period in my life as the relationship was conducted secretly and sporadically, with a lot of hurting on both sides as a result. We both felt totally isolated as lesbians, although a lot of our contemporaries must have known what was going on. Because of the secrecy and self-doubt, the relationship was doomed from the start. My partner subsequently returned to men while I remained celibate until we both left university and went back to women!

I wanted to give relationships a rest and took the opportunity to go abroad for a year to study at a foreign university. There, I felt more isolated than ever because I was in a country where homosexuality is completely underground. However, it was a period when I was totally 'out of circulation' and had space to consider what I really wanted. I joined a feminist group who, as far as I knew, were all straight.

I had always kept my brother in touch with what I was up to, so he knew about my first lesbian relationship. Because of its haphazard nature and my occasional relationships with men, this could not be termed an 'official coming out'. I had also told my best friend about my sexual confusion but she didn't really understand the implications; it was very strange to her.

Funnily enough, it was abroad, when I was sexually inactive and in a context of illiberal traditionalism and heterosexuality, that I began to come out, first to my landlady with whom I had developed a close friendship and then, on impulse, to my feminist group who were ridiculing lesbians. I felt totally depressed after coming out to this group and thought that they would totally reject me. I was surprised to find that, although they found it strange and not unfunny, they were fairly supportive, and I even discovered afterwards that one of their number was also a lesbian, living in a country where admitting to being a lesbian was akin to announcing that one was from Mars!

I take no pleasure in living a secret life and keeping my lesbianism a secret has always been a burden to me. I come from a very close family. I have never come out to my thirty-eight-year-old brother since he is very family orientated and ridicules gays, nor to my father because I was too frightened; he is now dead.

When I came back to England after a year abroad, I was more convinced than ever that I wanted to live a lesbian life. I began a relationship with the same best friend who had not understood my lesbianism, and at that stage I began to work up to telling my mother. It was very difficult as I feared being rejected, but in the end it wasn't as bad as I had imagined. She said that, although she was surprised, she was not shocked. It took her a long time to accept, but now she is fond of my girlfriend, and gets a lot of support from us emotionally.

I have come out to most of my friends. I try to avoid those people with whom I would not be comfortable in coming out. I have come out at work when my workmates have ridiculed gays. I tend to keep quiet unless someone is being anti-gay. I would feel terrible about not defending myself and pretending I was one of them. I do feel that, if absolutely everybody who was gay came out, there would be an ideological and sexual revolution in this country. I don't come out to my mother's friends to protect her as she lives in a very close community where gossip is rife, but I think it would be a very good thing to do for the sake of gay liberation. I wouldn't bother to come out to the milkman, for example. It doesn't seem relevant or worth the aggravation.

I think I have chosen a line of work which is independent of others, in the world of entertainment where attitudes are a bit more liberal than in the 'establishment'. I believe that being out at work would lead to problems for most people and I would never blame them for keeping quiet about it. I feel a little resentful that some avenues seem to be closed to me precisely because I have stopped myself from pursuing a career in the mainstream.

It is often easier coming out to young people because the older generation are often not at home with discussing any kind of sexuality, let alone homosexuality. But, ultimately, most people will have to bring themselves to accept this important aspect of a person's identity. We all fear rejection, but one can always tell oneself that people who don't accept us are not worth it anyway.

My personal situation with my family is unusual in that my mother is widowed and recently lost one of her children. It would be quite ridiculous for her to reject me as I am her only source of comfort and support in an incredibly sad situation. Parents who do reject their children because of their homosexuality are choosing to lose their living children and are totally incomprehensible to someone like myself and my mother who have experienced a real loss which we were not in a position to choose.

ANNA

Coming out for me was actually really easy. While I was straight or bisexual (though, come to think of it, I was never really bi) I was still just sharing a house with a man, but at that period of my life I was mixing a lot with lesbians. They were great; scarcely one of them pressured me. So one day, without any hard work or guilt or heart-searching, I just realized that I too could be one of that wonderful band. That, instead of just hanging out with them and admiring them, I could be one too. I only thought about it for about a week. My best friend didn't want me to, she said she'd lose me. Well, when she went up north with her bloke and had a baby, I knew she knew what she was talking about.

The first thing I did was to put up a notice in my local women's centre to try and get somewhere else to live. I started the notice 'Emerging lesbian . . .'. I like to think that I was the first person to use that term. It was 1980, maybe 1981. After that I started a lesbian support group which lasted four years. That was my family all that time. When it folded I was devastated. When I told some lesbians I'd been friendly with, they all said things like 'What took you so long?' and 'About time'. I had a lot of support back then.

It was a wonderful period, those first few years. I was often in love and often in terrible pain, but I felt at the time I'd done the best thing in the whole world for myself and berated myself for not having 'seen it' sooner. Looking back on my life then it seemed full of great and brave women who still believed in revolution. I think I'd just caught the tail-end of something that has changed, if not died. I'm very happy that I had that experience and wonder what has happened to me since then that has stripped the joy from my life.

GRACE

I haven't ever come out as such. Where I am half-way out it has been in the course of getting on with things, incidental rather than deliberate. I have never come out as an individual, except to my girlfriend, and then only after she came out to me first. It's a kind of inertia. I don't make any effort to come out, but I don't make an effort to stay closeted either.

I have not told anyone at work that I am gay. I can't see myself offering this information unasked for, the whole idea is too embarrassing. But I have to admit I have had opportunities to come out which I let slip by, like when a colleague asks what I am doing at the weekend, and I say I'm running a stall at a jumble sale, I could have said it was at the Gay Winter Fair but I didn't. And I could come out by wearing gay badges, but I have seldom done so and when I did nobody appeared to notice it. Once when I wore a Ken Livingstone badge one woman said, 'You're a Ken Livingstone fan? There's just one thing I don't like about him . . .' and I thought, if it's his support for gay rights then I'll have to say something, but she went on, 'It's this IRA business, they're just murderers'. I was half relieved and half disappointed that I wasn't going to have to defend Ken's gay rights policy. I wouldn't attempt to defend his IRA policy; besides, the woman was Irish so she knows more about it than I do.

Years ago when John Saunders lost his job in Scotland for being gay, I wrote an article about him and sent it to the local NALGO newsletter. The editor telephoned me to say she would print it, but it wouldn't be in the next edition as that would be devoted to the annual conference. As it happened the newsletter ceased to exist shortly afterwards and the article never did appear, but I would have been glad if it had and would have been ready to argue the case with anyone at work. A couple of years ago we all got a note with our payslips saying that our employer intended to become an equal opportunities employer, giving a list of grounds on which they proposed not to discriminate, the usual – sex, race, religion and so on, but not including sexual orientation. I wrote to the secretary of the committee which had been set up to work out the equal opportunities policy, pointing out the omission and enclosing some NALGO leaflets about gay rights at work. She wrote back, saying she had passed the leaflets on to the committee, and a few months later we got another note saying that the equal opportunities policy was now in force, and this time sexual orientation was included as one of the grounds for not discriminating. Probably they would have got around to thinking of it without my prompting, but I like to think I helped. It's not exactly coming out, though.

I have never told any of my family that I am gay, but they know I have been living with my girlfriend for seventeen years so they must have some idea. I have no relatives in England, the nearest are in Glasgow and I hardly ever see any of them except one aunt who comes to stay for a few weeks in the summer most years. When she is here, in order to have the time to entertain her, we cut down some of our political and social activity, but not altogether. We have taken her to a Gay Sweatshop play, an August Trust lunch, a Gay Authors Workshop reading, several Gemma meetings, an event at ULU at the end of a Gay Pride March; we couldn't take her on the march because she is seventy-five and her knees are not up to it. Also we have introduced her to many of our gay friends, some of whom are very outspoken. So, we think she must know by now, but she never mentions it, so neither do I.

I have taken part in gay pickets and petitioning locally, and have written numerous letters on gay subjects to the local news-paper, giving my real name and address. The editor is anti-gay and, every now and then, comes out with some absurd editorial opinion which needs replying to. They usually do print my let-ters, although sometimes in a garbled form, but this is one of the hazards of writing to newspapers, there is nothing one can do about it. All this is more 'out' than going on the anonymous Gay Pride March, though I do that too, of course, but I have had very little comeback.

At one time a local youth used to shout 'Gay liberation' at me whenever he saw me in the street, and one time I heard him arguing with some other youths, he telling them I was gay and they expressing scepticism. Once some children followed me down the road talking in loud voices about a gay television programme. Once I was in a lift in a high-rise block in Plaistow with two drunken men, strangers to me. One of them peered at my badge and read slowly 'Gay Vegetables'. 'Vegetarians,' I said. He looked puzzled and read it again, 'Gay Vegetables'. Then he said, 'Are you gay, then?' I said 'Yes', feeling a bit anxious and

wondering how much damage two drunk men could do to me
before the lift stopped. He said, 'That's all right. Everybody's
got to do what they've got to do'. I regularly read *Capital Gay*
openly on buses and the underground, so far no reaction from
other passengers. But none of this is really what is meant by
'coming out'. I have so far been lucky enough not to have much
contact with the police, my GP or public officials. I certainly
have not told any of them that I am gay, nor will I unless asked
a direct question, in which case I will tell the truth.

Why haven't I come out properly, by telling people straight
out instead of leaving it to be implied? I am not entirely sure. It
seems to come down to sheer embarrassment. I was brought up
to think it is not nice to talk about sex at all. But it is all right
in a political context. It is only now while writing this that it
has become clear to me. I had not bothered to think about it
before. I realize I feel an inhibition against discussing sexuality at
a personal level and can only do so as a generalization. I do think
I ought to come out properly, and I hope that eventually I will
overcome these feelings of embarrassment. I don't feel it's important to me personally, but politically it is important that everyone
who is able to come out does so.

MORAG

It is almost fifteen years since I first approached the gay scene
and started to live a gay life. I must be as far out now as it is
possible to be without wearing a badge – I'm not radical or a
particularly political person. If the subject comes up or my own
sexuality or marital status is asked about I usually tell the truth,
though the words used depend on the questioner and the situation. I don't lie . . . ever.

So, being out is important for me on two main levels: so that
I don't have to lead too much of a double life, and so that I am
a visible gay for all those who aren't particularly anti-gay but
who assume gays are 'someone else', say a poncy pansy or a
diesel dyke, who may exist in a gay ghetto of straight people's
imagination.

It is now so much an open part of my life and personality that
I couldn't retreat back into the closet if I wanted to. The more
times you're honest, and the longer you go on being honest, the
easier and more natural it becomes. I usually feel quietly confident

that the item of news about me will be well received. So much depends on how you answer the question or how you put the subject. I'm not radical, I'm not a crusader. Usually when the subject arises the listener isn't all that interested. They say 'Oh?' Sometimes they say, 'You're not, you're joking!' I assume that's because I don't look like their mental cliché of a dyke, and also they don't expect just to come across a gay woman, just like that, at work or on the bus.

I present myself in any way that seems relevant. I'm fairly articulate and present a calm, matter-of-fact approach, or maybe I'm witty and make a joke. The main thing is not to clobber the innocent listener or make them feel embarrassed or ignorant. For example, you don't say, 'Are you stupid, don't you know I'm gay?'

A lot of people ask a lot of questions; often 'Where do you go to meet other gays?' (the ghetto thing?) and 'When did you first know you were different?'. They usually reveal their views and ignorance on the subject by the form of their questioning. It's usually no major concern for them – why should it be? – but they are fascinated or intrigued and if I can answer their questions that's a bonus. I often say, 'No, I don't mind answering as many questions as you ask. I'd much rather you got the answers from me than from a book written by a straight psychiatrist, or that you believe the trash you read in the papers.'

At work I hope to get established and integrated *before* coming out. That sounds like a contradiction, but if you go in proclaiming you're lesbian that's *all* some people will ever see. In my present job, which I've held for two and a half years, I came out very gradually and gently to one or two people after almost a year. They knew me well by then and had some respect and liking for the way I do my job.

Sometimes you half hope the selected few you've confided in will gossip and spread the fact to save you the tricky task. Sometimes they do and the most unlikely colleagues and boss know, though *you* don't know they know! It can be tricky and perhaps uncomfortable if you're in a crowd of colleagues, half of whom know and half who don't. It leads to some farcical sitcom jokes and *double entendres* but could cause some of them embarrassment, which should be avoided. After all, it's my 'problem', not theirs.

I'm proud of how I've been able to handle the situation in this present job, but also proud, and often surprised, at my friends and colleagues and how low-key and matter-of-fact and okay they are.

I came out to my parents about a year and a half after I'd left home and moved quite a long way away. I'd fallen in love with a straight friend who knew and didn't mind, but who could not respond that way, and I was lovesick and heartbroken because she was leaving me to go back to university. I was so self-centred and naive that I never imagined the bombshell it would be to them. I've never gone through all the *Angst* and despair and soul-searching of other gays who have nervous breakdowns and make frenzied suicide attempts over realizing they're gay. I've been lucky. The news to my parents was that I was brokenhearted and blue, *not* that I was gay. . . .

That really illustrated my attitude, I suppose. People, the media, and so on, tend to say so-and-so is '*a* lesbian', although they would, if necessary, describe a straight woman as 'heterosexual', not '*a* heterosexual'. They imply that gays are labels and just that label. So I try not to say I'm a label. I was gay, but in that situation, my love was for another woman, that was the fact.

Anyhow, my parents were stunned. My dad never referred to the subject as such. My mum called me every filthy name under the sun and virtually disowned me: 'I only have one son and one daughter' sort of stuff. 'I always knew there was something not quite right about you.' Over the years she gradually accepted me and my being gay but, very much, I think, because neither my brother nor my twin sister, Megan, agreed that I was filth and to be shunned. They, and their spouses, always accepted me and their loyalty impressed my mum. Also, gradually, my mum (and dad?) realized that I hadn't got two heads or become a stranger – I was *still me*. I hadn't changed, I'd shifted perspective in their eyes, in one part of my identity and being.

I think when you do come out to your parents and family you have to accept that however much they then, or later, come to terms with it, they will still find it tricky to refer to your gayness with your aunts, uncles, grand-parents, close family friends, and so on. Nothing prepares them for describing your gay lifestyle. We, ourselves, never knew whether to refer to my 'friend' (twee!) or my 'lover' (racy, but a shade unserious?).

So, how do mums and dads cope? I wrote to my few relatives so that the job was done and most are okay, if noncommittal.

My favourite two aunts were decisive and positive as I'd hoped and would have expected. Another uncle did his boring duty as a vicar to 'pity' me, but he does keep in touch. His dire prognostications came true when my five-year relationship ended!

The further out you come, the more people you eventually have to tell, else it becomes very complicated.

The most unlikely people accept the revelation calmly. Others can be surprisingly naff and ignorant. My rather old-fashioned, unsophisticated sister-in-law actually made what I think to be a valid moral judgement before my sister's first marriage split-up. She'd been seeing an older, married guy and this was really frowned upon by my sister-in-law who compared it to my being gay. 'Well, whatever Morag is doing,' she said, 'she's hurting no one and not breaking up a marriage. It's something between two unattached adults.'

My mum, initially, rather dwelled on the unnatural nature of two women in bed together. I often use the comparison when people say they just can't imagine fancying someone of their own sex, by remarking that hetero love scenes on television or film really turn me off, especially if the woman is gorgeous (what a waste!). The thought for me of going with a guy – I did have two or three male lovers many light years ago – is just as repulsive and really does seem *unnatural*! Well, it isn't natural for me. It is quite a complex battlefield, dealing with family, but I personally am relieved I told them so soon and before it became a big hurdle.

The negative side, with some straight friends, is that although they accept my gayness (and why the bloody hell shouldn't they?!) it's of very little interest to some of them and I can feel rather dismissed and diminished. If I refer to a girlfriend, their eyes go a bit blank. If I'd got a boyfriend, I suppose their own empathy would make it a bit more interesting for them, but it's just as important to me.

My closer colleagues all care, but also I care back and, being a bit older than a lot of them, I'm something of an older sister or agony aunt to them. I care and can offer advice to them about their boyfriends and so on. Neither they nor I find that strange or impossible. I suppose they've got an insight into someone being gay, and it's mostly being much the same through the actual real-life, everyday me . . . being in love and exuberant or heartbroken and hurt is the same for all of us. 'Love is an emotion, not a gender', as the drag-queen remarked in *EastEnders*.

There are acres of experience and feeling where any fellow gays can sympathize. It is good to be in a gay bar or club among your own kind, but I'm grateful I can mix in either gay or straight company and take just the bits I want from both.

I make my mates laugh with the more comic side of being gay. They like my own self-acceptance, I suppose, and my involved-but-detached attitude. For instance, if my lover and I wanted a set of bath-towels saying 'Hers' and 'Hers' for Christmas, we'd just have to swap with a male gay couple who had a set the same colour of 'His' and 'Hers'. And you go into a male gay couple's bathroom and there's two shavers, or two boxes of tampons in a lesbian couple's bathroom. After a hasty session of lusty undressing you grope on the floor and pick up your lover's bra by mistake, and it's too big or too small and ridiculous!

If all this is presented as just matter-of-fact it can be fun and entertaining and much more educational for 'ignorant' straights. If they all go on about fancying a film star or a rock star, I just refer to a *female* star *I* fancy. Oh, yes?

The more serious issues do get touched on, but possibly sink in less well. They see me as well-adjusted and friendly and that's diplomatic in itself. A major misconception I've done a little to combat is that awful myth that lesbians hate all men. A lot of questions are about that sort of thing. It all does some good. Some of what I discuss is general, the rest personal and particular to me. Of course, we're individuals. I do wish, if only for one day or for one hour, every gay would stand up and be counted, visible and proud! It would amaze us, let alone them!

I have been abused (verbally!) and shouted at and the like, but nearly always by strangers. When someone actually knows an individual they can accept the 'odd' bits. I'm not a label and I won't hide. I'm a rounded human being who happens to be gay. That's the tale I tell.

6

Mind and body

LAURA

With the aid of retrospect, I can now recognize my lesbianism as being a part of my life from an early age, exhibiting itself in 'tomboyishness', in interest in and fear of girls, in disinterest in and jealousy of boys (for their status, what was 'given' them, and not for anything *inherent* in the male), in deliberate attempts to fit into the accepted norms while clearly not doing so, and in a desperate kind of loneliness, despite the fact of having three sisters, including a twin. I cannot remember not feeling different.

But retrospect does not reveal 'as it was' and the aspects listed above do not simply relate to my sexuality, with or without self-awareness, but to my whole emotional being. I had come across many images of homosexuality in literature, though almost none specifically about lesbianism. I do recall reading D. H. Lawrence's *The Rainbow*, in which I found the lesbian scene exciting and, therefore, frightening; it is also, there, clearly unnatural and so cannot survive and nor, of course, does Ursula want it to survive. Lesbianism is seen by Lawrence as something that 'has no life of its own'. Literature was where my life was lived; that is, not in the actual world and not, somehow, connected with me. I had no consciousness of my own emotional reality; that was too frightening a thing.

A very close friend at school had told me he was gay. I was initially shocked (envious?) but came to like and admire this, but I could still hold it away from myself. I eventually found myself at university with gay women and men friends but *nothing* bore any relation to me; I was totally closed off from myself. I liked gay people. They were 'positive' images, but I was totally ignorant of my own sexuality and utterly, utterly screwed up.

Traditional education, even in literature, was neither enlightening nor supportive. Attitudes have changed a little now: there is a patronizing, kindergarten 'know-your-place' admission of literature's little sister – women's writing (always optional courses); in a provincial university in the sixties and early seventies a course was created, directed and taught by men and largely for men. I have no quarrel with male artists, male audiences and male teachers *per se*, but it seems women must seek for an equilibrium without the support of the establishment which may, ultimately, be a good thing. In nineteen years of full-time education I learnt next to nothing about myself or my sisters except, of course, how men saw us. Education is a highly restricted and restrictive concept.

The only thing that was becoming clear during my time at university, whether I liked it or not, was that sex with men (I did try!) terrified and appalled me; the one clue I had to myself, to my sexuality, was that my earliest sexual dreams were lesbian and incestuous. I couldn't put my dreams into someone else's book or life, they were mine, and they didn't present me with the most acceptable life-plan I could have imagined. For obvious reasons, I couldn't or wouldn't talk with any member of my family; I was incapable of talking to anyone at all about myself. The only place I was getting was a crash-dive into alcoholism.

Never in touch with myself, not relating even to those images I liked, and destroying myself with fear and alcohol, I 'naturally' found myself sitting in front of a psychiatrist – a straight, male, almost old-enough-to-be-my-father, progressive and rather wonderful psychiatrist. My academic tutor, who was male, had sensed I was cracking up, not sleeping, not talking, drinking heavily and really living in a state of terror and aloneness. My university tutor, female, had made the appointment for me to see the doctor who was usually entrusted with 'problem cases'. He was, naturally, fatherly, and we had fortnightly talks in addition to the sleeping pills and minor tranquillizers he prescribed me. There was a kind of charming naivety in all this, as well as a genuine concern which provided some support. This same doctor was also notorious for ascribing most problems in women students to 'boyfriend trouble'; he eventually got round to this topic, but when I said I wasn't interested in boyfriends he dropped the subject. At the time, that was all I had allowed myself to know; it was a further six years before I could say I was a lesbian.

When the extent of my drinking was discovered (a minimum of half a bottle of spirits a day), the treatment became a little more serious. Overnight I moved from being a student having some difficulties to a potential, if not actual, alcoholic who was probably depressive too. When questions regarding my sexuality arose I usually skirted round them or joked; again, if I was trying to hint at my own confusion, it wasn't being taken up. I can't recall being aware, or it being suggested, at any point during this period that my sexuality might be relevant to what I was going through, let alone that it should matter! I continued to see the doctor fortnightly, which gave me the excuse for not going home in the vacations, and to be prescribed stronger sleeping pills and stronger tranquillizers. Since I was continuing to drink as much, if not more, my doctor realized that I was killing myself. He referred me to a psychiatrist who had just opened a clinic for the treatment of drug and alcohol abuse.

I consider my experience of the psychiatric world one of the luckiest breaks in my life. I have seen more than enough on both sides of the fence. Besides having two two-year periods of treatment, I have also worked as a psychiatric social worker for six months. Not surprisingly, I have also met many in the gay world who have had psychiatric treatment and many who work in the caring professions. As a result, I know that the positive treatment I received is very, very rare in the public health service. My first step into that world could so easily have been the first on a downhill slide into institutionalization.

I was fortunate to find myself in a relatively enlightened set-up, a climate in which feelings, self-respect and trust were valued, and in which one was encouraged to confront and work through difficulties that were sometimes so blocked off that only by opening up to an extreme of vulnerability could one begin to become conscious of them. What, in retrospect, now seems remarkable, is that both in individual and in group psychotherapy there was very little attention paid to sexuality: in therapy, as in almost every social situation, sexuality was an awesome and fearful subject. Some allowance should be made for my own blocking of the subject. I wasn't aware at the time of a 'gap'; and I do believe my psychiatrist was 'pacing' me, maybe both of us. For example, in my in-patients group, during three months of hospitalization, there was one man who, after several weeks of the ten-week course, disclosed that he was homosexual. He was in his late thirties, a teacher, and found it extremely painful to tell us about his homosexuality. He had not been able to come out to his parents. The therapist and I encouraged him to confront his feelings about his parents in relation to his sexuality, as everyone else seemed to shy off. As he struggled to speak his head began to corkscrew away from his body, and he was helpless to stop this. His parents were literally screwing him up and tearing him apart. He failed, in the end, to speak with his parents and, not long after, he killed himself. At no time was anyone else encouraged to relate what was happening to this man with their own sexuality and, after he had gone, sexuality, as opposed to 'trouble with boyfriends', disappeared from discussions. No one, including staff, was prepared to go along with what he was trying to do, which meant acknowledging the central and absolute importance of his sexuality.

While in hospital I found myself, and there weren't other words I could use for it, falling in love with the woman who was a nurse-therapist for our group. My psychiatrist knew it, she felt it and I, if wordlessly, had to acknowledge it. This was not explored, it was allowed to be, and I don't mean just 'tolerated'. None of us, I can now see, could confront the simple fact of that emotional commitment although it was recognized; I had to live with it and learn to value my feelings or dismiss a vital and intense part of myself. The real lesson, apart from that of realizing that to give up on my feelings was to give up on myself, I learned through all this during the five years it took to work through was that the professionals in the psychiatric field are only human and often as frightened of looking at sexuality, of seeing its potential complexity, as the vast majority of people. If you are lucky, they have discovered their own weaknesses and are prepared to admit them to a degree which allows you the space to be. In more traditional institutions, where the assumption of authority and theory on the part of the professional 'expert', usually fully endorsed by the 'patient', who rarely understands there is a choice, displaces the need for the acknowledgement of such weaknesses or vulnerability, I would have been categorized as sick. In my case, I shall be eternally grateful for the support that helped me reach the understanding that I am responsible for my feelings, and that those feelings are all right.

The first time I made love with a woman, at the age of twenty-six, was terrifying! However, frightened and confused as I was, and here I think I am quite lucky, I knew from the first that this was right, and that I had made a choice in that act that I couldn't move back from. I was still trying to fit in, trying to be heterosexual, but the intense struggle this created in me meant my finally seeking help and seeing a psychologist, again male and straight, for a further two years. The difference now was that I was making choices and decisions for myself. I knew that I needed support to work through this; by myself I was slipping back into old, destructive patterns. I could select that help. I, briefly, saw one psychiatrist who, probably in response to my pointing out the sexism in his questionnaire which asked if I had any difficulties with relationships with the opposite sex, clearly saw that my 'problem' was that I thought I was lesbian. I didn't think this was a problem. I saw learning to accept and enjoy myself, not getting a 'cure', as the process ahead. Fortunately, he was not able to take me on, or I would have rejected help at that time.

Discovering my lesbianism was a growing process leading to the liberation and acceptance of my 'self', including my sexuality, and ultimately being able to embrace that larger self with joy. I do not think that there is an end to such a process, for I continue to grow within, and beyond, loving relationships I have had and have. I have been happy in my sexual expression as I have learned to love, and not to ignore myself which is more than, but inseparable from, that sexual expression.

DOROTHY

Depression. The grey demon. The cold voice at the river's edge, saying, 'Jump'. The razor's edge that gave me scars. A two years' possession. I needed help, I got family therapy. I spit on the memory and the gap in my head it's made, a big black block of lost time I cannot, except in the briefest of moments, remember. Leaving home and loving women released me from the dead spell, and only when friends die does its sleeping miasma cloud my spirit. I see the funny side these days. It's the best weapon.

MAXINE

My first experience of lesbian sex was with Gaby, and was wonderful. It was eighteen years ago now, and I can still tingle from
the memory! It wasn't a momentous big decision or anything.
We were always sleeping over at her house as she was an only
child and we worked part-time in the same shop. So sharing
baths and cuddles just turned into lots more. We knew better
than to broadcast from the rooftops that we were in love, but
we didn't know enough to feel guilty or have hang-ups about
doing or not doing whatever we felt like. For a while, one of
my boyfriends was a man who managed a garage and I spent six
months with him having sex in phone boxes, under cars, on the
football terraces, his idea of a big turn-on. As far as I was concerned, that was sex – you open your legs and wait for the grunt.
What I was doing with Gaby just didn't have a name and didn't
need one. I suppose it's odd that we never really talked about
what we were doing, but at the time it didn't seem like that.

I really encountered lesbianism as a word when I encountered
feminism. I left home when I was eighteen and encountered all
sorts of exciting ideas and ways of doing things that I'd never
come across before. My first relationship with a woman after I'd
left home wasn't a very good experience, though. She called
herself a feminist, too, but luckily there were enough other
women around to show me that there were as many types of
feminism as there were women with that label. Carla was physically and emotionally abusive both in and out of bed, and at
first I just accepted it because I thought, 'Well, this is a sexual
relationship and if ones with men are like that, why shouldn't
ones with women be?' After a while I got involved with my
local Women's Aid group, though, and began to realize that I
was being a bit two-faced. While I was with Carla I got raped
twice, both times by men who thought that was an okay way
of saying they were personally offended by me being a dyke. I
went a bit loopy after the second time, which Carla couldn't cope
with. So we had a very flamboyant parting of the ways!

I started coming to terms with my sexuality and labelling
myself for people more often quite soon after I left Carla. I saw
three male therapists on the NHS, one session with each, who
all saw my lesbianism as my main problem and had various
theories, like I was being loopy as a way of dealing with the

guilt at having enjoyed being raped. The therapist who said this was sexually turned on by me being a lesbian, and I got a definite impression that after a few more sessions he'd have been offering some experiencing cures! I told them where to get off, which I'm very proud of now, because I was just about at the most powerless and shot to pieces I've ever been in my life. Friends helped me find a feminist therapist. She was, and still is, straight, but is now a good friend and she did me a lot of good. As I got more involved with feminist things, I also got to meet lots more dykes. Funnily enough, though, it was coming across all these positive images that opened my eyes to all the negative ones. I think being raped was part of that process too. Although I can look back on my relationships with men while I was living at home and call my sexual involvement with them rape on some level, there's nothing to compare with the absolute terror of some man you've never met before overhearing your conversation in a pub and being underneath him in an alley ten minutes later. I think the viciousness of both these rapes will be with me for ever and ever. One of them had a knife and I really thought he was going to kill me just because I'm a dyke. I don't think I can communicate how unbelievable that is, or what a perfect way it is of making a woman feel like a piece of shit.

I got raped another time (I've heard all the jokes about being careless, thank you) after both of these, and of course it was horrific and took some getting over, but it wasn't the same somehow. I don't think I can explain, but there was something about that third time that it was me as a woman, which is just something I am. But the other two times it was about my sexual choice. I know it wasn't really, I've worked as a rape counsellor for six years and I know all the stuff about why men rape women is because they know they're allowed to. The time when I got raped outside the pub, though, I just know it wouldn't have happened if we'd been talking about flower arrangements, or about our boyfriends. There's still a big part of me that finds it totally unbelievable that I'm living on a planet where that can happen.

I think one thing that I do now that I probably wouldn't be doing if I hadn't had those experiences is that every three or four years I sleep with a man friend. I spend a lot of my time being scared of men and sometimes it gets to the point where it's hard to function in a city which has a lot of men in it and my fear of being raped again gets to take over my life too much. So I sleep with someone safe, always someone I can trust enough to turn it into something to laugh during, but I always give myself a hard time about it afterwards. I don't know if some of that comes from all this stuff about lesbianism being second-best, the 'you haven't met the right man' stuff. I know that being with women isn't a gap-filler for me, but it just seems to help me function in a man-made world to have some controlled sexual contact once in a while. End of justification!

I make a point of making sure my GP knows I'm a lesbian, but when I get a new doctor I ask her not to write it on my notes. This is partly because my aforementioned loopiness involved convincing the police that I wasn't a dyke (it's very complicated and I'm not going to explain!) and although it was a long time ago I still get fears sometimes that they're going to come and do me for lying to them! Mainly, though, I use my dykedom as a test of whether this is a woman I'm happy to have as my GP. If she can't cope I go and find someone who can. One of the times I got raped I was left with pelvic inflammatory disease and, when I have a recurrence of it, it comes out as infections that are often heterosexually transmitted. I get less assertive than I usually am when I have to deal with it, though, and I want to know that I'm not going to get all that crap about whether my boyfriend's been sleeping with the neighbour's dog when I go for treatment.

I love being a dyke, I love being with other women and laughing and living every bit of my life with other women, and most of the work I do is about caring for other women while caring for myself too. It is a choice though. I don't believe in biological bases of behaviour, particularly as men use these 'explanations' to let themselves off the hook for all the shit they get away with, and I know that if my life had happened differently I would have married one of the men I was seeing to cover up my relationship with Gaby, or got pregnant and panicked into straightdom, or succumbed to everyone's expectations to be a wifey. Even when I think of all the ways we get punished for being a dyke, though, I'm fucking glad I didn't!

ISABELLE   (*written in 1986*)

Why do you mention AIDS in a directive called *Lesbians and Health?* AIDS has nothing to do with lesbians.

VIV   (*written in 1986*)

I was first advised to see a psychiatrist when I was fourteen or fifteen. I had an accidental drug overdose which was labelled 'attempted suicide', which it definitely was not, and all such cases are automatically referred to a psychiatrist. In fact, I did not get to see him and had no contact, personally, with any kind of therapist for several years after that, although I have suffered from depression since childhood. In a way I administered my own treatment to myself instead, since for ten years I regularly took drugs and, for two years, had a heroin habit. When I did stop using heroin every day I went to see a private psychotherapist who was a lesbian too, recommended by my homoeopath.

When I was nineteen I started psychiatric nursing and spent about a year as an auxiliary nurse in a large hospital, general and psychiatric. I was always in the closet at work where the attitude was extremely heterosexual. In fact, one of the reasons I gave up nursing was the anti-lesbian attitude of a lot of nurses, not expressed to me, personally, since they didn't know, but in general conversation. It made me uncomfortable and unable to express myself at work. I know one or two gay male nurses. One tried to come out at work and was told by his superiors that if he didn't keep quiet about being gay then he would never be promoted. Nursing is such a hierarchy that, lower down the scale, gays have to be very careful. No doubt, higher up they are known and tolerated, but only when being 'discreet'. It's particularly hard on lesbians as it's not exactly a 'butch' job. It can be better for gay men as in a predominantly female environment they get more tolerance from their co-workers. As far as patients go, I only remember one, and he was an alcoholic. His medical notes mentioned he was homosexual but as far as I know it didn't affect his treatment; again, it was largely ignored. But the whole hierarchical and patronizing atmosphere in hospitals, in which patients are allotted the role of children with the nurses as their parents, means that it's hard to assert oneself as an individual even if heterosexual, let alone homosexual.

As far as AIDS goes, it's relevant to me in several ways. Several gay male friends are HTLVIII* positive, although none has yet developed the syndrome. I expect it is only a matter of time before, by the law of averages, one of them does, and this worries me. The attitude of the media to AIDS and the way that they try to use it to whip up hatred of gay people bothers me too. Although it's mainly against gay men it crosses over to cover gay women too. Because I have been an intravenous drug-user I have been at high risk of catching the virus. Last year I was quite ill, some of the symptoms were similar to HTLVIII symptoms, and for a while I was worried that I was HTLVIII positive. I went to the Special Clinic to be tested. I know all the considerations about whether to test or not to test and so on, but I wanted to know. In fact, I wasn't asked whether or not I actually agreed to the test, nor given counselling or advice, just given that test among others. The attitude of the doctors and nurses at the clinic when I told them I had been a junkie and that I am a lesbian was non-judgemental and polite at all times. I turned out to be negative. They stressed several times that I did not have AIDS, and suggested I had some other virus which they could not identify and could not treat. Obviously, it was a relief to be HTLVIII negative, but stressful to think I have something which diminishes my health. Since I came off heroin two and a half years ago my health has been constantly bad, and I also have glandular problems. Although I still occasionally use heroin I rarely use needles and, if I do, they are clean, so I know I won't get the virus that way.

However, I am constantly at risk of sexually transmitted diseases as I work as an escort, a polite term for prostitute. I always insist on my clients using condoms where possible, and keep a sharp eye out for AIDS statistics and information, who and where the new cases are. As far as I know, it has not yet appeared in the prostitute community here. The prospect of its doing so is worrying. If, and when, it happens I would then have to consider giving up my job, or adopting stringent safe-sex techniques with virtually no contact at all. At the moment my safe-sex techniques consist of a short discussion on hygiene with my client, do they have regular check-ups, where have they been recently, do they realize the need for safe sex, and so on, and insisting on condoms.

* Later renamed HIV.

I also try to ascertain if they are bisexual, in which case I would be insistent on minimal body contact with them, with no exchange of bodily fluids. My other option, should AIDS appear among working girls here, would be to specialize purely in non-direct-contact sado-masochism; in other words, set up as a dominatrix. Ironically, this, the safest method of working from our point of view and the least likely way to transmit any STDs, is the most heavily penalized by law. Working as an escort I am extremely unlikely to be arrested and charged. Working as a dominatrix I can be charged with running a disorderly house and risk a likely prison sentence. This last point outrages me.

I suppose AIDS is thus almost as relevant to me as to any gay man, in the personal sense. In a general sense it concerns me anyway, as it may affect my friends and does affect the gay community of which I am a part. I am appalled by the backlash in the States, but try to take the positive attitude that, for every reactionary around, there is a well-informed, reasonable person with a sympathetic opinion. The States has always had more extreme extremes than Britain, so I don't think it will be as bad here. I also think that people don't believe everything they read in the papers. I've just heard that the hospice for AIDS patients in West London will be going ahead, despite much opposition from public and press. I see this as a positive sign of more tolerant attitudes. Eventually, AIDS will not be so concentrated in the gay community so more time will have to be spent doing something about it rather than inciting homophobia. I don't think women are seen to be as much of a threat as gay men. Lesbians are never taken seriously. But, broadly speaking, anti-gay feeling affects lesbians generally.

ROSE   (*written in 1990, in response to a directive on the lesbian-gay divide*)

Why do you say, 'Perhaps lesbians might care to say how they feel about AIDS even being mentioned in this directive'? AIDS is our problem too.

7

Together

SUSAN

I have been involved in a lesbian relationship for eighteen months. It is a monogamous relationship by mutual preference. Before Maureen and I became lovers I had slept with one other woman, who I knew well as a friend, when she was on a weekend visit to me. I did not feel for her as a lover and our sexual relationship ended then, though the friendship is still strong.

Our relationship has not always been easy, but the difficult patches are by far outnumbered by the good times. Occasionally, we joke about getting married, which I see as a way of expressing a commitment to each other in a non-threatening way. The idea of having our relationship blessed is meaningless to me, as formal religion of any kind is irrelevant to my life and to both of us. In any case, the permanence of a union of two people can never be fully assured; I would rather say that I am committed to her for the foreseeable future.

To suggest that long-term relationships between gay people ape the heterosexual model strikes me as very negative. It denies the existence of emotional needs and desires that everyone has, regardless of their sexuality. Not all people want to fulfil these needs through a monogamous relationship. Some have many sexual partners, concurrently or consecutively, some prefer monogamy, others are celibate. Many take all of these paths at different times of their lives, but what they choose is not necessarily dictated by their sexuality; other influences, such as the attitudes and activities of friends, are present as well. I see gay relationships as an opportunity of breaking away from heterosexual stereotypes. For myself, being involved in a lesbian relationship means trying to establish and maintain a truly equal partnership, with both of us taking responsibility for matters emotional and practical. This is easier with no existing stereotypes to challenge first, such as 'who wears the trousers' or wields the dishcloth. Of course, there are stereotypes about lesbians, both outside and within lesbian culture, but I wonder to what extent these are imposed by or absorbed from heterosexual society which can see gay culture only through straight eyes. It is possible that straight friends of ours see one of us as the 'masculine' partner and the other as the 'fem' one, but the issue has never arisen and the people concerned have not, I suspect, confronted their own prejudices.

I have not had any negative reactions from friends about being lesbian, though I am unsure of a few I have not seen since I came out. There is no direct pressure from my parents; I just know they don't approve. My way of coping with that is not to talk about my lover with them, which I do not like myself for but hope that sometime I will be strong enough to be more relaxed and open about this whole part of my life. I do feel a general pressure not to reveal my sexuality, especially when I am with people I don't know well. So there are times when I refer to Maureen only as my friend rather than my lover, whereas if I were involved with a man I would feel quite easy about calling him my boyfriend. Again, I hope that as I become more confident as a lesbian I will feel less inhibited by society's conventions.

I have not felt compelled to make any changes in my behaviour as a result of our relationship. What I do sometimes find a problem is that Maureen smokes and drinks heavily, so that I find it hard to stop smoking completely and I drink more when with her than when we are apart. However, in the words of the women's movement, that is my choice! The most necessary change in my life is that I travel more now, as we have lived a hundred and fifty miles apart for most of our time together.

On the question as to whether it is possible to have a complete and fulfilling life without a partner, this depends a lot on the ability of the single person to seek and obtain emotional satisfaction from friends rather than a lover. When I have been single I have not felt less fulfilled in my activities, rather I felt free to do what I wanted, whether that involved cooking the evening meal or moving house, without always having to think about a lover's wishes. Yet I do not feel restricted in my choices because of my current involvement. It is another consideration if I have to make major changes in my life, but I would not let it stop me doing something I felt was important for me. Sometimes I feel lonely, even though I live with people I know well and am close to. When I was single I sometimes felt lonely and unloved, despite knowing that I had close friends. At times I feel frustrated that Maureen and I cannot live together because our jobs keep us in different parts of the country, but once that low point is over and I am involved in my life here, that frustration ceases to be overwhelming and I can feel more self-sufficient. In general, I feel that everyone has an infinite capacity to continue finding out about themselves and what they need to feel 'fulfilled'. This increasing self-awareness varies according to one's friends, work and so on, and whether one is involved with a lover. Such a relationship is not the only way to personal development. The general attitude that being half a couple is surely what everyone wants is, perhaps, the hardest image to overcome for people who, by chance or choice, are single or celibate or both.

I cannot predict whether Maureen and I will always be together. I cannot take for granted that I will always be 'married' or assume that I will have children to look after me in my old age. At present, aged twenty-five, I have no fears about being old and lonely. When I think of retirement, I imagine living with other 'right-on grannies', sharing a flat with like-minded friends as I do now. That vision may change as I get older, but I would certainly not want to get married or have children to insure against a lonely old age. That seems rather a lot to expect, as a partner may die before me and children might not want to know me by then.

Sex is important to Maureen and me; we both want it and enjoy it. I like the intimacy that it entails and creates. The desire for sex varies; some of our weekends together are very passionate, other times we are more platonic. At the start of our relationship, we would make love a lot; now that that initial euphoria has died down, sex is more fulfilling and relaxed. In fact, it just gets better and better! There are times when Maureen is in the mood and I'm not, in which case either one of us gives in to the other's mood. Sometimes, when I really don't want to make love, I feel guilty for 'failing her', but this issue has never caused problems for us. If I am honest, I have to admit that my lack of desire is sometimes more to do with laziness than anything else.

My feelings about multi-partnering have indeed changed over the last few years. I realized, after several attempts, that I got no pleasure from one-night stands or casual affairs. The best sex for me has always been in the context of a monogamous relationship, which I think is the consequence of the trust that takes time to develop between two lovers. I came to realize this before AIDS. I do not know how much less I would have experimented if AIDS had been generally known about at that stage of my life, for going to bed with someone is not always a careful and considered move. But my awareness of AIDS, together with my increased self-awareness, will make me more careful in choosing future sexual partners or sexual activities.

Jealousy has not featured in our relationship, apart from one occasion when I was very strongly attracted to one of my male flatmates. I did not mention it to Maureen, so as not to hurt her, and hoped the situation would resolve itself without her being involved – and without sleeping with him! However, she realized what I was feeling and was hurt by it. She confronted me about it, which quite shocked me, but I realized I could not lie to her because she would see through me. The fact that a man was involved was especially hurtful to her and was also a shock to me. I had, rather naively, supposed that, now I knew I was a lesbian, I would never again have sexual feelings towards men. This incident actually strengthened our relationship and established the basis for greater honesty with each other.

I think that, in this case, my lover was quite justified in her jealousy. I was being dishonest, for though I loved her I was abusing the trust she had in me and in the relationship by not admitting that I was attracted to someone else. The commitment that had been to her alone was confounded by the feelings I had for the man. As I do not go in for 'open' relationships, I was beginning to feel that maybe I didn't love her.

A last word on monogamy. I do sense a personal move towards fewer sexual partners and more long-term relationships, both among media-hype and among my own friends. I cannot tell which has the greater influence on the other side. But, at the same time, there are still many people who go in for non-monogamous sex, despite the risk of contracting AIDS or other sexually transmitted diseases. I think the attitude that casual sex is okay and desirable will not disappear easily or quickly, nor is it an attitude exclusive to one particular age group. After all, the wheel cannot be disinvented.

PAT

At the moment I am in a long-term relationship; well, I consider it long-term since it's lasted two years so far, though it's showing signs of cracking now. It's the longest relationship I've had – I'm now twenty.

I've enjoyed being part of a steady relationship. I do think there's something to be said for the monogamous relationship, although it can feel very restrictive. Being tied up doesn't stop me fancying other women or regretting lost 'chances'. In my relationship I don't know if it would strictly be called mono-gamous. In reality it is, but it's open in theory. I don't worry overmuch about loneliness in old age; it's a long way off. On the other hand it would be nice now to have someone to come home to, to reproduce the security of my own family; things like having a cuppa waiting for someone when they come in from the cold, watching telly together in the evenings and so on. I like security and routines like that. My present girlfriend has com-pletely different ideas, seeing such things as bourgeois and as necessarily involving oppressing one partner.

We met via Gemma. We'd written to each other for about a year before we even met. I was just getting over breaking up with my first ever girlfriend. We were both at school, in the upper sixth, and we ended up writing twenty-page letters to each other every week. Anyway, eventually she suggested we meet; this was after we'd both left home for further education. It was pretty well decided between us that, catastrophes apart, we'd have a relationship, and lose our sexual innocence together. I suppose it was a bit weird really but we both wanted a relationship and were prepared to work at it.

We slept together very soon after meeting as a result, which was a pity in a way because we ended up getting close afterwards, rather than getting close first. At the time I was very lonely in my first term at university and she was insecure too, and I think we both wondered whether, if we didn't do it that weekend, we might never meet again.

I don't think I adjusted my behaviour to suit her, nor vice-versa. We're very different people so we tend, and always have

tended, to clash a lot. At first our politics matched, as did our
taste in films and books, but we've both changed a lot since then,
so we've not that many shared interests any more.

Sex was the area with which we had the greatest trouble. After
all that bilge about lesbians just doing it naturally, there we were
not getting anywhere. It was really discouraging. I'd had some
sexual experience, mostly in the back seats of cars, and in nooks
and crannies of school and that had been really great. Of course,
I assumed that sex would always be like that, but there just
wasn't any spark between us for ages. Our first night was a real
disappointment to me; Marilyn still doesn't know this! There was
a lot of cuddling and cossetting, which was okay, but very little
genital contact. She'd not ever had an orgasm when we met, and
still only comes if she uses a vibrator for ages. Maybe that's why,
but she's never given me an orgasm manually, and I really miss
that. On the other hand I guess I tended to shy off sex for ages.
She was really intense and I began to feel as though, if we ever
cuddled, that was it, she'd expect sex. This lasted for about a
year and a half. In the last six months or so the sex between us
has really started to come together, though we rarely come unless
we – how shall I put it? – see to our own needs towards the end.
Typical, that just as the sex gets good we start to break up!
Nowadays I guess our sexual appetites are fairly equal. I don't
feel like she's mauling me continuously any more and so I'm
much more responsive myself. It took a hell of a long time for
that to come about, though. From all this, you probably think
that we never talked about sex together, but we did . . . oh god,
did we? I think we've got just about every sex manual on the
market between us! Talking, demonstrating what we needed and
so on, but the trouble was neither of us could really appreciate
the other's feelings for ages, because we're so different. She likes
direct, hard touching; the mere thought just makes me cross my
legs and start working out my shopping list. I was always frightened of hurting her, and she was always too rough for me. Still,
it worked out, more or less. I don't know why our sex suddenly
started getting better, it just happened.

Even when it comes to doing things the other wasn't interested
in, we vary. I'm really into water sports. For a long time that
was just a non-starter. We talked about it, but the idea really
turned her off. On the other hand, she discovered a mild interest
in sado-masochism during our first few sexual encounters, some

of which bores me. Tying someone up takes so long that any interest I felt tended to wear off; ditto dropping wax onto someone. As for biting someone's breasts, yuk. Mostly, though, we were quite experimental. We talked a lot about what interested us, or what we'd like to try, and usually had a bash at it at some stage. I've never let her tie me down, though.

As for pressures outside our relationship, my parents were no trouble. Once they could see that we were steady girlfriends, they just accepted it and they really like her. In a way that is itself a pressure, though, because they assume that we'll always stay together, live together and retire together to somewhere in the countryside. When we break up I should think they will react much the same as they would to my sister divorcing, or my brother breaking off his engagement, with bewilderment and sorrow. Marilyn's parents don't even know that she's gay. I've met them, spent a visit with them. They think I'm just a nice, innocent (that is, not man-mad) friend of their equally innocent daughter. My mates have accepted her. I don't know what they think of her as a person, but they accept her as my bit, in the same way that I'd accept their other halves without necessarily wanting their boyfriends as friends, apart from that link. Marilyn's chums are all gay or lesbian, anyway. They've not put any pressures on us at all.

Marilyn has just got a council bedsit so we've somewhere to be together. When we were in our first year at college she was in lodgings so I couldn't visit her and she had to stay in my room in the college. She had no hassle from the other girls in my residences; they all knew I was gay and referred to her as 'your friend'. We did have some trouble with the university cleaners though. There was a little-publicized rule which said that if you had someone to stay the night in your room then you had to book them a camp bed. No one knew of this rule, and no one would have wanted to hire them a camp bed, anyway. The cleaners didn't report any of the hets in the block for this activity, but reported me to the accommodation officer for having a woman in my room for dirty activities without hiring her a camp bed. I was crapping myself in case I was thrown out on my ear, and really furious. Anyway, the accommodation officer was really nice about it. She told me that there was this rule, and she was quite aware that the cleaners only enforced it selectively, but to shut them up it would be better if I hired a camp bed in future;

whether or not we used it was up to us. This upset Marilyn who saw it as the first in what might be a long stream of persecutions.

In my parents' village I've had an egg thrown at the window when Marilyn was staying with us, and the little brats tend to yell supposed insults like 'lezzies' at us as we toddle about. This scares Marilyn, but having grown up in our reputedly peaceful village I'm relatively acclimatized to such things. We do show affection in public to some extent, linking arms as we go about, and kissing in alleyways. It irritates me that Marilyn is so timorous about this; she seems to fear that little old ladies will come and heckle us.

I wouldn't say we suffered from jealousy at all. We're quite open about our little infatuations. The only time I got a bit worried was when she began to talk about a close lesbian friend of hers, because that was more serious.

Another area on which we differ is marriage. If marriage was open to gays then I would probably like to be married eventually. I don't feel the need for a blessing at all. I'm a secular humanist and run a mile from the Christian church. On the other hand, it would be nice to have some sort of ceremony whereby you could mark your intentions 'in the eyes of the gay centre' maybe. And, besides, we miss out on all the toast racks as things stand.

On the whole I'm not sorry at all that I've had a long-term relationship. We've been to a lot of places, and explored the London scene together. The two years we've spent together have had their troubles but there have been great moments as well. We rely on each other. After the first six months you get to believe that she's there for you; she listens to your problems and worries; she's the only person I'm honest with about my failures. On the whole, I like to pretend not to care about such things, but when you've been with someone a long time you can talk about such things. Also, when there's something bad happening you've got a private source of comfort and support, someone to take your side against the world – we only argue in private! – and someone to make an early cup of tea for.

GRACE

I think monogamy or non-monogamy is a matter of personal choice and there is no 'right' or 'wrong' way of life. We should follow our own inclinations and not try to impose our views on others. If attracted to someone whose views on monogamy are very different from one's own, I think it is best to back off and not let a relationship develop, because trying to change the other person to fit in with oneself or trying to change oneself to fit in with the other is unlikely to succeed and the failure could cause a lot of misery.

My own inclination is to monogamy. I don't consider this to be copying anything. Rather I think that there is an instinct among humans to form pairs, that some people have this instinct very strongly while others have hardly got it at all, and being heterosexual or homosexual has nothing to do with it. But I think gender might have something to do with it. It does seem from observation that women are more inclined to monogamy than men (though, of course, there is a lot of overlap) and age too might affect it, young people being more curious and experimental. I am in two minds about the changes that are happening now. On the one hand, I rather welcome any trend to monogamy because I think for some people it is not so much a restriction as a release from an imagined obligation to be non-monogamous. At the same time I feel very angry towards the moralists who have eagerly taken up the AIDS issue and made it an occasion for preaching against gays and non-monogamous hets. They reject safe sex because they see it blurring the edges of the moral issue and it might even permit people to go on enjoying themselves. It looks as though some of them would rather see people be put at risk of AIDS than be informed about safety, and that seems to me to be really immoral.

I think it is possible for some people to have a complete and fulfilling life without a partnership, if they have the strength of mind to withstand the constant battering of pro-marriage propaganda from family and the media. I can't say I have noticed a difference between people in long-term relationships and others. The difference is rather between people who are content with their state and those who are not. One woman of my acquaintance is bitter and resentful of lesbian couples, and I am sure this is because she would really like to be part of a couple herself. Another woman who says cheerfully that she couldn't live with anybody is friendly and relaxed with lesbian couples, because she is happy in being single. I think the prospect of loneliness in old age is something *everybody* should be prepared to face up to. Those in long-term relationships should be aware that they might outlive their partners, and even having children is no guarantee. I used to visit a woman in an old people's home and one of her fellow residents was a widow with six children, none of whom ever came to see her.

DEBORAH

My first long-term relationship lasted a period just short of five years. We met at work in the police service where, for many reasons, we had to be careful of our behaviour towards each other. We were good friends for about twelve months before the relationship started. I had been lesbian for a number of years at that time. She had had one fairly short-term affair with a woman already in a long-term relationship.

I have had many 'one-night stand' type meetings, but must admit that the most enduring and satisfying affairs have been based on an initial friendship rather than pure physical attraction. We lived together in a house which I was already in the process of buying when we met, and consequently moved, yuppie-like, into a larger house, which I also bought. Yes, I subsequently became very poor when the relationship ended and I became responsible in full for the upkeep of a two-income home.

I was not then, nor now, aware of any behavioural changes caused by that relationship. I think, because I was very young at nineteen, as she was, that we both matured as a natural process throughout the time we were together.

My last relationship ended two years ago. I was aware during this affair that my behaviour was changing rapidly in accordance with my lover's covert demands. At this time I had become fairly active in a semi-political way, was out totally to family and friends and was positive regarding my sexuality in the sense that, although I was unemployed, I would not actively hide my life-style. My lover was in the closet, everywhere. I willingly went along with the depoliticizing of my life, believing at the time that I could only function with a partner. I feel that this relationship was unequal in a lot of ways. I accepted these inequalities as I had, shortly before, suffered a bout of depression which made me quite dependent. This relationship had its foundations firmly rooted in what I would now term negative areas: sex, emotional dependence, economic dependence and intellectual starvation. The relationship would have died a natural death as I left our shared home, her house, to go to university while she went to work in Saudi Arabia.

I have chosen to write about these two relationships because my position was all but reversed regarding the equity within the partnerships, but they ended under similar circumstances, different to others where the affair petered out or I made the decision to end it. In both the above relationships my partners formed new relationships while still partnering me. This, in itself, is acceptable to me as I have never really had a wish to be in a monogamous relationship, but find that all too often the other 'flings' take your place in your lover's life.

This is my second period of celibacy which has lasted over twelve months. I feel that I can live without a partner in the typical sense, and use all my energy to support women friends, lesbian and heterosexual, and homosexual men. My political consciousness is well and truly raised with regard to areas relating to gender issues and equal rights. I have very ambiguous feelings towards having same-sex relationships blessed or even legalizing marriage. I say this because the partnership I mentioned first was actually blessed by a closeted gay priest who was a friend of a friend. This was not of great importance to me, but to my partner and her family. On the other hand, I feel that a commitment between two people *is* between two people and surely does not need legitimizing, regardless of your sexual orientation. The whole idea of marriage smacks of possessing and being possessed.

I have noticed a great deal of difference over the past five years or so relating to the behaviour of acquaintances in long-term partnerships. It has become like some exclusive club. I mean that in the sense that many of them (un)intentionally exclude non-partnered people. The shift in their support is amazing. Having been close, supportive, active women, they have become enthralled by the material gains possible in a two-waged house and are now, in many ways, less concerned with fighting for equal rights. I suspect, and I have been guilty of this myself, that if the relationship ends they will realize that the world is totally geared to couples and instantly run off to find themselves another half. This is not intended to sound arrogant, but is a general observation of what I see around me more and more. I have fallen into the trap on many occasions, hence my celibacy which acts as a safeguard against me falling in lust and making commitments by default. I feel I need to know what I am capable of before I enter into another partnership, as when I am in love my behaviour pattern changes dramatically. That is, when I am actively in a sexual and emotional relationship I am able to give emotionally to the same extent to friends on a non-physical level, and feel that spiritually my friendships are more important than having one person providing physical, emotional and spiritual support. It has taken me, and I am still learning every day, many years to realize that I cannot cope with the intensity of such close relationships. I do not like the feelings that totally encompass me and the dependency I feel.

I will not deny that the thought of spending the rest of my life alone is unappealing but, and it is a large 'but', I do not feel capable of handling all that goes with a committed long-term partnership at this time, mainly because I have little time to devote to one person in that sense and would come to resent someone who diverted me from my current long-term ambitions. Rationally, I realize the choice would be mine, but you know what it's like when the heart starts to rule the head . . . disaster! If I do spend the rest of my life without a partner I do not feel I will regret it or feel my life is wasted. Often my most lonely periods have been within a relationship.

A special area of any mass-observation programme is the 'day-diary', when volunteers are invited to record everything they can of a given single day. The following two passages record Christmas Day, 1989.

ROSEMARY

I spent all day in bed coughing, due to a flu virus, waited on hand and foot by my mate who had had it a little earlier, but was still coughing. Luckily we had two different coughs, she sounding like a trombone, I like a cat being sick. I ate a very little vegan food, drank lemon and fizz, no alcohol, feeling too grotty, lots of aspirins and Strepsils. Watched television now and then, atrocious programmes, no Elvis film yet again. I wrote an aggrieved letter to the BBC. Read Dickens as he is the best author to read when ill, he just flows along, *Martin Chuzzlewit*, and fell in love with the way Jonas is written. Might be the flu virus but I see *Martin Chuzzlewit* as one of Dickens's gay novels like *David Copperfield*. If you want my flu-ridden ramblings, here they are: Jonas, murderer and wife-beater, is beautifully drawn, his S/M courting of Merry is especially fine. Though Dickens keeps telling us what a rotter Jonas is, yet he somehow dwells on his physical presence with what I can only call tenderness. I think *he* was in love with Jonas. A bit rough. Jonas marries late, and for money. He tells his wife if he had to choose again he would not marry but would keep with his friends, the gaudy bunch of crooks in whose lives women are conspicuously absent; even when they have a party it is all men. Montagu Tigg, the most gaudy of all, accuses him of wanting to 'jilt' him by going abroad. All the language around Jonas is passionate and physical, even his suicide isn't Dickens's often maudlin treatment of death, but is raw and real. The other repressed homosexual is, I think, Poll Sweedle-pipe, 'Polly', lone, unmarried and elderly as Dickens says, who at the end adopts the irrepressible monkey of a boy, Bailey. Well, what is that all about, eh? 'Uncle seeks nephew', *Capital Gay* ads, I should say. Bailey is to work with him in the business and inherit his all.

Xmas Day, then, was spent in bed. We have a double bed we practically live in now we have the television on the chest of drawers opposite. The kitchen is immediately next door so we have all our meals in bed, read, write, sew and the like there. As I had barely enough energy to wash myself, my mate did all the work of the day, feeding us plus our two cats and three or four visiting cats. I didn't phone anyone and nobody phoned me, thank goodness.

Mate cooked dinner, her delicious chestnut and mushroom pie which we always have for a treat at Xmas. She is Xmas-mad, the flat is dripping with tinsel and streamers, this bedroom looks like a Hindu temple, and we get masses of cards, mostly from gay friends. She is not Xtian but the carols and hymns blare out as she really revels in it all. I am trying to, but I'm rather anti-Xmas really as Xmas Day was a day of gloom in our family; my father hated it and did his best to make it a day of misery; my mother, being religious, tried to jolly it up, so we had these two opposing forces battling it out, and the shadow of the marital war games still hangs over the twenty-fifth for me, though I am trying to get rid of it. A gay Xmas is nicer and less trouble.

We like to have this day to ourselves so we can stay in bed, ill or not, and play with our presents and watch television or listen to the radio or read. The lesbian friends are invited round on the twenty-third usually, and the gay men on the twenty-

sixth; never the twain shall meet. And we are the pair who
oppose separatism! But we don't want aggro at Xmas, and someone might say something silly to someone of the opposite sex
so, at the gay men's party, we only invite those few women who
can handle men as well, for example the odd bisexual.

GRACE

Listened to the Queen's speech on BBC2 at 7.35, noted she was
wearing a nice festive colourful dress for a change, not her usual
style. Hoped she was going to get through the speech without
mentioning God, but she failed. Watched *Brookside* and *After
Henry*, then telephoned a gay man friend, disguising my voice as
a drunken Scotsman and enquired if there was 'ony chance of a
bit of leg-over the night'. In a cautious sort of voice he said he
thought it very unlikely. I then sang 'We wish you a merry
Christmas' and invited him to come for a drink and Christmas
cake tomorrow afternoon. I think he was relieved I was not really
a drunken Scotsman after his body.

Watched Alf Garnett on TV then gave cats their Christmas
treat of chicken roll and made toast for my girlfriend but did not
want any myself, having unwisely stuffed myself with nuts and
Maltesers. I went into the lounge and sat there a few minutes
with the light off, and the Christmas tree lights on, admiring the
effect of the coloured lights and the decorations and thinking
about what I might do tomorrow, that being another holiday,
and how I ought not just to idle the time away eating and
watching television.

I really like Christmas. I always expect to enjoy it and I always
do, even if I am a bit ill as seems to happen sometimes, no doubt
because of the time of year. I love the music and the tinsel and
glitter, the feeling of excitement in the streets and the shops just
before Christmas, and giving and receiving cards and presents. I
don't know how people can dislike it or feel depressed by it.
Even if you have no money it is still free to walk in the streets
and look at the Christmas lights, hear the music in the shops and
see the shop assistants with tinsel in their hair. I am not a religious
person but I do not find any contradiction in this. If I had to
justify myself I would say I am celebrating the winter Solstice
and the return of the sun.

LAURA

The needs and reasons underlying relationships are probably as many as relationships themselves. But perhaps there is some justification for generalizing about the theory of lesbian relationships and the changes in that theory we have witnessed over the past fifteen years or so. The importance of early feminism is loosening the ties of heterosexual models and demanding sexual liberation is evident in the enthusiasm with which non-monogamy was embraced in the late 1970s. What I suspect was really happening, however, was that the force of a women's movement to a degree lifted women out of the immediately personal, pushing individual relationships temporarily into second place, sisterhood before self. I am not interested at this point whether this might be thought of as a good or a bad thing, only that this is how it seemed to me to be. Since then, I am aware of two processes, which might in fact be inseparable. The first is that feminism has clearly lost that sweeping energy that can lift and carry women along, committing them to a movement which makes them look outwards rather than inwards. The second is that those women who were a part of that stronger movement have now grown older and perhaps are shifting away from the need for a collective process towards an awareness of existing for oneself, still within a larger world, but recognizing that being together with oneself is a necessary basis for strength.

At the same time, our environment has radically changed. We have moved from Wilson's to Thatcher's Britain where self-seeking and self-serving are the order of the day. If you don't put number one first, then you don't come anywhere. Private revolt cannot touch Thatcher's philosophy; to survive in any kind of alternative mode to Thatcher's you need support as well as inner strength. For reasons of health, national politics and economics, it does not surprise me that more lesbians and gay men seem to favour long-term relationships, if not necessarily rigid monogamy, today.

So much for some theory, which is a lot easier to formulate than looking at what you do in or with your own life!

For myself, I don't believe there is such a thing as an entirely rational choice between a long-term relationship or not. My first fully lesbian relationship, in that by that time I had come to terms with being lesbian, was forever, but isn't that always the case? I moved in with her. We put up bookshelves, decorated a new bedroom, went to dinner with her mother, and so on and so forth. Only, I wasn't allowed to grow. Everything was wonderful to begin with, so that's how it should stay. It was a type of psychological bondage. After six months I left. Later I realized that what I'd really needed was endorsement and consolidation of my sexuality; that achieved, I had to move on. That may sound hard, but for me it underlines the idea that what I need from a relationship, that is, when need is a dominating factor, will dictate the style of that relationship.

The next two years were a continuation of that consolidation, largely played out on 'the scene', with quite a few fairly brief (some *very* brief!) liaisons which were often fun, but never really satisfactory. As you head towards the age of thirty you begin to wonder if you *can* fall in love! So, naturally, it happened. I fell in love, and it was going to last forever. About four months to be precise. And I was devastated as she took off with a woman whom I'd hardly noticed but who was very cheerfully butch. My only grim satisfaction was grasping what was happening without being told – ten out of ten for sensitivity. I hurt like hell, but in the end what I was aware of most was the intensity of feeling I'd experienced at every stage; that I couldn't regret any of it because above all else was the fact of my being fully alive, feeling right through from outrageous joy to almost intolerable pain. That is not something I can experience through brief liaisons; for me it is something that comes only with the love and trust that allows me to reveal and experience my vulnerable self, my feeling self.

This kind of intensity necessitates commitment, and I see myself as an essentially monogamous person; this is not to say that, while I am involved in a long-term relationship, I am not aware of and attracted to other women – it's just that I'm very unlikely to do anything other than enjoy that awareness and appreciation. This is not a moral stance: a relationship which allows you fully to experience your feelings is likely to open you up to a much larger and exciting emotional world which is there to be enjoyed.

But to get back to reality, as this is beginning to sound like a bed of roses, which it is – roots, thorns, aphids and all!

I first met my lover when she came for an interview for a volunteer post at the place where I work. At this moment in time I know of one other dyke in our immediate locality, so I needn't go on about meeting like-minded people and the rest. Fiona knew where I stood from the start; I wasn't into being discreet about my choice of ear-rings or badges. I did not know where she stood apart from her being something of an awakening feminist. For four months we were on a basis of quite friendly, but slightly distanced, good relations. It was only when she gave me a black triangle that something finally clicked! But this interlude, I think, was a good thing. As it was we were both, I felt, rather frightened of what was beginning to happen, but there was reassurance in having known each other for some time. And as soon as we really spoke to each other we became lovers.

Ours is not an entirely conventional relationship because, for nineteen out of the twenty months we have been together, we've been over a hundred miles apart and only see each other for two or three days every fortnight. This produces its own pressures. First of all, it was 'obvious' that we should live together, and that Fiona would come to me as I had the steady job. This put her under a terrific strain, and therefore our relationship too, because she felt, rightly, that she had a lot of exploring to do. Our relationship wasn't and isn't the entire world. It was the oblique forms this pressure took that brought us both, at about the same time, to realize what was wrong. We then did exactly the same thing in reverse, that is, that I should move in with her. Eventually, we came to understand that we were trying to fit into a model which, to date, is not appropriate to our situation, though there is naturally a desire to be together more than we are.

Living so far apart has meant that we've avoided many of the difficulties that couples meet, and also the traditional heterosexual trap of the one becoming subservient to the other. We realize that such an arrangement does have advantages. It also has a lot of frustration and for me emphasizes my isolation within my particular community. I am certainly accepted and tolerated here as an out lesbian and have met actual aggression on only a couple of occasions in the nearly four years since I moved here from the city. However, I do not have a lesbian community. My focus is with my lover who then becomes friend, counsellor and, sometimes, not-so-willing sufferer for all my difficulties and needs, as well as lover and sharer in joy.

Further, for the second time during our relationship, I am

trying to be a sober alcoholic with her support, for my own sake as well as for the sake of our relationship. This, for Fiona, is beginning to mean a re-examination of her attitude to alcohol and therefore will necessitate a self-exploration which, I feel, she finds a frightening prospect. But this is very much something that she feels she needs to do. She is also some years younger than me and I know, at times, she asks herself why things are like this, and whether she really wants it. These are thoughts that also frighten me. It is intense, and can be exhausting.

But, though we have both, separately, sometimes tried to walk round difficulties, we have both found that it doesn't work for either of us. Still, talking immediately about something which is clearly wrong is often extremely difficult and painful. I think we are both guilty, at times, of believing that we should get things right. Recently we have been considering finding or creating a 'third party', perhaps a therapist or therapy group, because we are beginning to see that we don't have to be a perfect couple so that heterosexuals can't point to us to show 'it's all wrong' and 'it can't possibly work'; we are only human, we don't have to isolate ourselves. We have something that is worth some pain if necessary, but we don't have to torture ourselves.

Well, that's what I'm saying and thinking and believing, and telling myself it's not all on my side. Possibly my worst fault is my shortfall on self-love and that can be very punishing for my lover. The adjustment I have to work at is acceptance of, and respect for, myself. That'll be doing us both a favour.

As in other things, in sex I seem to be the more needing partner, but we have a good sexual relationship and I think we know each other well enough for there not to be misunderstandings. Those there have been have always involved alcohol, but it's taken me a long time to begin to come to terms with that. In less literal terms, there is always a sobering process after the first heady days and nights of loving; but this is to do with growing ease and confidence, and trust in each other, less need and more loving. I feel that we are continuing to explore each other and ourselves without the desperation that comes from wanting to possess and be possessed.

Without being exhibitionist, we are openly affectionate with each other; if we are not, there's something wrong between us. We are both out with our families and Fiona has met my twin sister and her husband and my mother. I haven't met any of her family yet. I think I can say that everyone behaves in a very civilized fashion, and the least said the better. I do feel hurt by this, the continuing hypocrisy, but it could be worse. Undoubtedly, we are both most relaxed with friends, not all of whom are gay, and I have always been delighted to introduce my lover to friends and other lesbians. I would not dream of trying to keep her away from others as if she were some kind of property. I have only felt truly jealous once in my life, and that was years ago. I was shocked to realize it. It seems to me that anger or sorrow are much more appropriate responses to situations which might be supposed to inspire jealousy. Everything may be a risk, but guarding against possibilities is a waste of energy. It was harder for my lover when she first introduced me to her new lesbian friends after she'd moved. It was the first time she'd been in that situation and it was rather testing.

I would not opt for the single life. I *think* I could handle it but I would know that, for me, some vital part of my expression would be missing. I invest a great deal in our relationship. Sometimes I fear it might be too much for it to bear, but we've come through so far, albeit with tears as well as joy. And we both keep changing and growing, which is living. And so our relationship is living and developing too.

JO

I don't know at what age I became aware of homosexuality though it must have been before the day I saw Tom Robinson on the telly singing 'Sing if you're glad to be gay'. I must have been about fourteen, which seems awfully late, but homosexuality just wasn't talked about in the small town where I grew up. I really liked the song and agreed with it. It just seemed logical to me that love was a good thing and why should it matter who or what it was directed at? So, being a serious young Sagittarian, honesty before all else, I joined in singing with him. Not very surprisingly, though it was to me at the time, my mum asked me if I thought I might be gay. I said 'No', but it did get me thinking. There was nothing in my morals against it, but being gay was something people outside our town did and something that *men* did. I think I decided I was bisexual within five minutes of my mum asking me if I was gay. After all, if she'd asked, there was a possibility I could be. I don't think I had either a positive or a negative image of homosexuality. It was something 'other' and, as such, as both intriguing, exotic and a bit scary.

It wasn't until I moved to the city when I was sixteen that I met anyone who was out and gay. I was going around with people involved in one of the theatres and they had male friends who were gay. There were five of us from sixth form college who went round together and our local was the gay pub. By this time I'd got involved in my first sexual relationship with a man I'd met on an archaeological dig during the summer, but since he was working two hundred miles away that didn't interfere with my life much. Although I never talked about my involvement with the gay scene with him, a couple of years later I heard a rumour that he'd made sexual advances to a man on a dig. I don't know about the truth of this but most of the men I've been involved with have had a certain amount of homosexuality. I don't know if this is to do with the sort of men I'm attracted to or just men in general!

So, at this time, my social life was centred around the gay scene. The atmosphere at the time was one of experimentation. I don't think all adolescents go through a homosexual phase but I think most go through a phase of sexual and emotional experimentation and, if the circumstances are conducive, this may well include homosexuality. Although I didn't really notice it at the time, it was the boys who experimented with homosexuality rather than the girls. This didn't stop me from telling a bisexual man I slept with that I wanted to sleep with women, though I later found out that he'd told my friends. This certainly didn't cause any problems for me since all it led to was a bit of gossiping behind my back which was heard by the woman who was to become my first female lover. I think it helped us get together.

I didn't start my first relationship with a woman until I was nineteen. I'd known her by sight for about two years. At this time I was very promiscuous, sleeping with lots of men as a way of exploring life and the different ways people live and think. I'd been working as an archaeologist for a year since dropping out of college, which meant a lot of travelling, but I was still based in the city. On one of these stays at home I became sexually involved with a man with whom my first woman lover had had a relationship for two years and was still a good friend. Me and the man used to go and see her quite often and, by the time I left the city again, me and the woman had got to the stage of seeing each other on our own.

While I was away we exchanged a lot of letters and in one of them she told me she was coming out as a lesbian. I wrote back and said I loved her, which surprised me then and still does, because it's not a term I use lightly and is something that, except with her, I only say after I've been involved with someone for a long time. When I got back to the city we got together, but the physical side was disastrous. We were both very nervous and unsure about how to go about anything. As we're both very verbal we could sort out our fears of being a same-sex couple (neither of us really knew any lesbians) but when it came to sex we were at a loss. Because lesbians don't tend to be very explicit about sex, all we came across in books was the general idea that lesbians are very good at it since, being women themselves, they know what a woman wants. Of course, this just made us feel more inadequate.

So, mentally we had a great relationship but physically I think we just ended up laying a lot of guilt on ourselves for not knowing how to do it properly. I think having been involved with average heterosexual men before didn't help, since you learn that it's not really up to you to take the initiative or even to think about what you want sexually. Our non-monogamous coupled relationship continued for two and a half years, but I think the 'not quite happening-ness' of the sexual side and the guilt surrounding it played a part in ending it. However, we're still very closely involved with each other and are both more confident about our sexual expression with women these days, and we've vaguely discussed becoming sexually involved again. For my birthday last year she gave me a copy of *Lesbian Sex* by Jo Ann Loulan and we sat and looked at it and said, 'If we'd had this book four years ago, we wouldn't have had half the problems we did'. I think the lack of lesbian sex education can be a big problem for women who want sexual relations with other women.

Strangely enough, it was sex with my last male lover that has given me confidence about my sexual expression with women. Since he wasn't into penetration and, for him, sex is about communication of love and not just gratification I had enough space with him to learn to be active and to be able to say what I wanted. I think the other main factor has been choosing not to sleep with men. My sexuality is bisexual in that I enjoy sex with men and women, but because our society makes it easier to sleep with men in so many different ways I've found I've needed to make the choice of only sleeping with women; otherwise, I don't confront and overcome my shyness and lack of confidence with women. Nowadays I don't think that I'm just not going to know what to do in bed with a woman because I know I do, but I still find it hard to know how to go about getting there. Still, I've had a bit of practice and that wasn't too bad – in fact, it was very nice – so I'm sure it can only get better.

I first started coming out to people in general when I was nineteen to twenty, but it's a continuing process, especially as I moved around quite a bit and people tend to assume you're heterosexual. I want people to know I'm not heterosexual, but it tends to be only close friends I keep up to date with shifts of focus along the lesbian–bisexual spectrum. Since I live in a separatist women's house and am mainly involved with women's things now, this helps people not to see me as heterosexual. I told my mum that I was very attracted to women when I was twenty but we've never talked about it. She's very ambivalent about our relationship which might have something to do with my homosexuality and it might not. We're certainly going to need to talk about it if our communication's going to get any better. Since I see my family very rarely I haven't told my sister and dad that I'm gay, but I'm beginning to feel more of a need to know that my life's less chaotic and I'm re-evaluating what my family means to me and my life. I can't see any of them being really enthusiastic about my sexuality but likewise I can't see them rejecting me on the basis of it.

(Since writing the above) my lifestyle has changed dramatically. About six months ago I started co-parenting an eighteen-month-old girl with a lesbian womyn who is not my lover. Around the same time I also realized that I no longer identified as a bisexual. Part of this was due to the fact that as a mother I have limited time for relationships and therefore less time and energy for working through the inevitable problems and oppressions of relating to men. Of course, preferring womyn was also a major factor.

I suppose I have quite a liberal attitude to relationships. I can see the value in everything from one-night stands to living with one womyn for the whole of one's life. I guess, really, I want to do the lot. Perhaps this comes from having Venus in Scorpio! In relating to womyn, I've had one long-term relationship and four casual relationships. The long-term relationship was non-monogamous and effectively lasted four years, although sex was only part of the relationship for two and a half of those years. The casual relationships lasted between one night and a couple of months.

At the moment I'm much more interested in a long-term relationship than a casual one. I want the learning and enjoyment of loving a womyn as we both change and grow. Perhaps I'm cynical but I don't really see long-term relationships lasting more than two or three years. I do feel it's possible to have a fulfilling life without a lover. Also, that if womyn can't live happily without a lover then having one is just a sort of prop. I think we do need lovers because there's bits of ourselves and others we don't see otherwise, but likewise we need to live some of our lives without lovers. Until this year I'd never spent more than a couple of months without a long-term lover and I've really enjoyed and needed the space and time I've had by not having a long-term lover.

For both my co-parent and myself our decision to parent together meant some serious thinking about relationships, what we wanted out of them, what we could put into them and how much time we had for them. We had both made a commitment to parenting our child that takes precedence over love relation-ships. Since we wish to live together without others at this time we don't have the option of living with our lovers. We may choose to live communally with other womyn in the future but feel we'd prefer not to have the strains and complications of a home life that includes lovers of one or both of us. Although we both have some regrets about not being able to live with lovers, we both have a strong need for stability and in discussion have realized that we actually have our stability needs better met by this arrangement than in the emotional ups-and-downs of living with a lover. It is important for both of us that we've not lovers for stability and also because, as womyn, lesbians and feminists, we're struggling against the patriarchy and its basic structure of the nuclear family. So what we're doing fulfils our political and emotional needs.

Of course, it's not all so simple. Co-parenting is such a big commitment of time, energy and emotion that it's a problem finding enough left over to deal with relationships. I only know two other lesbian couples who are co-parenting not as lovers. One couple used to be lovers and are now splitting up although continuing to live together and co-parent. Neither of the other couple has had a lover since they started co-parenting about nine months ago. All the other co-parenting couples I met at the lesbian mothers' conference this summer were lovers. From talking to womyn there I gathered that this tends to mean that the non-biological mother has little, if any, access to the child if the relationship breaks up.

Both of us have previously been committed to relating non-monogamously, although now it's doubtful that we'll have time for more than one lover unless we have casual relationships and neither of us is particularly into this at the moment.

My co-parent began a relationship four months ago and this has been a time of learning for all of us, especially since her lover had never had a relationship with a womyn with children before. It's sometimes hard for us all to keep everyone else's needs in mind. My co-parent's lover needs time for her own life, her other lover and her friends as well as spending time with my co-parent. Until recently communication between the two of us has been quite bad but we've done a bit of work on it lately and it's much better.

My co-parent, hereafter referred to as Gayle, needs time with her lover, her child and me and, occasionally, even some time on her own. I need time with my kid that feels like choice, and not just because Gayle wants time on her own with her lover, and enough time with Gayle to keep good communication going with her. Recently, I also realized I needed time doing fun things just for myself. I'd gotten so tangled up learning to parent that I'd forgotten one day I'd have enough energy left over to do things for myself.

Until now I haven't had a lover. I'm beginning to get involved with a womyn in the city where we will shortly be moving. This weekend we're going to a womyn's holiday house with my kid. Gayle said I needn't take our child with me, but I decided I wanted to because I need my lovers to be able to cope with me having a kid. Of course, I don't want my child always to be around when I'm with a lover. That's where a co-parent comes in handy!

At the moment we live in the countryside in Scotland, ten miles from the nearest town. We've only been here six months and within about fifteen miles we know about twenty dykes. We also have lots of womyn visiting and we go and stay with friends too. I know for many lesbians it's much more difficult, especially if they feel the need to stay in the closet, because it makes it even harder to meet other lesbians because they don't know you are. Both of us are very open. We dress peace-camp style which I guess gets us noticed, especially by the vast network of womyn connected with Greenham, many of them dykes. And amongst our jewellery are labyrines, lesbian symbols and badges saying things like 'Lesbian mothers are great'. We also get very little hassle. One womyn in the village has stopped speaking to us but the rest are fine, in fact, really friendly on the whole.

I don't see a long-term relationship as security in old age. I want enough honesty in my relationships for them to finish if it's time for them, whether it's been three months or thirty years. I think if I'm in a relationship when I'm sixty, but don't have a lesbian community, I'll still feel lonely. No, I don't feel equipped for being lonely in old age, who is, which is why, when my child grows up, I'll probably be putting some time into creating some womyn's land in the country specifically orientated to having older womyn as well as younger ones living in it. Then when I'm sixty or seventy or so I can go and live in a house there with a couple of older dykes with younger ones nearby into helping out if we needed it; occasional visits to and from lovers, family, friends, living with the land and, when the time comes, dying with it.

8

Power

GRACE

Soon after the London Lesbian and Gay Centre opened there was an article in *Capital Gay* about S/M Dykes being refused meeting space there. This enraged me so much that I wrote a very angry letter to the management committee, and a letter of support to S/M Dykes. They now have another place to meet so that particular issue is dead, but I still feel the same about it. It is clear to me that people who try to ban others from using the Centre are themselves seeking power over other people, and that this, if successful, would be power in reality, unlike the fantasy power of S/M games. I don't acknowledge the right of any pressure group to impose its policy on me. I regret the decision of any minority to boycott the Centre because it is a loss which weakens the unity of gay people. However it is their right to go where they please. It is not their right to stop others from using the Centre. If it comes to a choice between those who want to impose their will on everybody else, and those who want to do their own thing with other like-minded people, then my support has to go to the latter.

About dress codes: I don't like them. Maybe this is in part because when I was young there was nothing like the freedom of dress generally that there is now. People throughout all classes of society were expected to dress conventionally, with strict gender demarcation, and were judged by the way they dressed. I felt strongly that this judging by appearances was a shallow, superficial way of looking at people, and I value the comparative freedom we have now. Apart from the restricting effect of dress conventions in themselves, I am repelled by the motives of those who impose them, because people's clothes are a way of expressing themselves, and suppressing freedom of dress is an attack on the personality. That is what I think of dress codes, personally. Whether they should be imposed is another matter. The only dress codes I know of that actually exist are what I have read of men's clubs which stipulate leather and denim. I deplore this as silly and childish. However, I have to concede that how I feel about it is irrelevant, and if they want to behave in a way that I consider silly they have every right to do so. So, yes to dress codes in private clubs, mixed or single-sex alike, where the members have democratically decided in favour of them. I would only say that I think they should mention their dress codes in all publicity to avoid annoying or embarrassing visitors and potential members. But I feel strongly that LLGC and any other gay centres in other towns are a special case. These should be for all gay people to go dressed as they wish and be free from harassment by pressure groups. Gay people of unconventional appearance get hassled in straight venues and public places. We should be free from it in our own centres at least.

About intimidation: I feel uneasy in the street when I encounter groups of youths in skinhead or Rastafarian dress. I perceive both as a potential threat to myself and I could say I feel intimidated by them even though they do nothing to threaten me. It is to do with their being young and male, aggravated by what I see as an aggressive style of dress. But I acknowledge that this is my problem, not theirs. It is my responsibility to control my feelings about their appearance, and to assess the situation as it actually is, that is what they are *doing*, not how they *look*. It is not their responsibility to change their dress to suit me.

I have been a victim of violence. I was beaten up and my jaw broken by a man unknown to me in the street at night, for what reason I don't know, presumably robbery, but I had nothing on me to steal. This violence, where I was attacked and injured without warning and without my consent, has nothing to do with S/M. I am against violence, but where people consent together to use a measured, controlled amount of violence in the context of their relationship, that is their business. I have nothing to say about it and I have no right to say anything about it. Violence in self-defence is, I think, permissible because, although I may admire the courage of the person who refuses to be provoked and literally turns the other cheek, I don't expect everybody to be like that and I am not like it myself. The violence I oppose is the unprovoked attack on a person who has not sought it and does not consent to it.

I have tried to think through and understand the feelings of people who need violence to achieve sexual expression; I don't know how far I have succeeded. I don't share these feelings in fact, but I try to share them in imagination. I can imagine that, for some, consensual S/M is useless and they need to impose violence on unconsenting victims. These people need to be restrained for the sake of the freedom of the rest of us.

JO

The first time S/M came into my life as anything I spoke to anyone about was in 1983. I got together with my first womyn lover in late 1981. She was also bisexual and by early 1983, when she tentatively told me about her masochistic feelings, we'd already been through a lot together. Since we were so close, and what she was basically telling me was that she wanted to find out more about it by reading and talking about it, I wanted to support her in that. The fact that I didn't have any firm views on it helped, but also the fact that, at the time and, as far as I can tell, now, the stance of anti-S/M womyn seemed to be to suppress all information and discussion made me angry, as I felt and feel that hiding it all away isn't going to help anyone.

The summer of '83 I went to the Lavender Menace bookshop in Edinburgh and bought *Coming to Power* for my girlfriend. That autumn we both read and re-read it. Some parts of it made me feel sick and some really turned me on. What upset me most of all about the book was realizing how much of 'normal' interaction between people is sado-masochistic, all the little mind-games and so on. I think we all do things like ignoring people, withdrawing affection and being cold in order to show our hurt when others don't act as we want them to.

Reading *Coming to Power* made me realize that I definitely didn't want to do any of the more obvious S/M sexual practices although some of the role-playing mind-games did attract me to a certain extent. We dipped slightly into some of the role-playing stuff that winter and spring but never really got into it and stopped doing it altogether pretty quickly. I think we both felt uncomfortable with it all.

For the next year I didn't think about S/M at all, though quite a few womyn in the city where I lived read *Coming to Power* with pretty much the same reaction as us. I moved into lesbian feminist circles again in 1985 and S/M was definitely out. I still can't relate to the 'it's politically incorrect and gives lesbians a bad name' line, however.

When I started living with and co-parenting with Gayle I found she was very anti-S/M but it comes from an 'it makes me sick' point of view, which I can relate to much better, and which made me start to think about what I felt. I'd known for quite a while that I knew the lines both sides took but couldn't make my mind up and then I started listening to my own reaction from wanting to know who I am and not which camp I'm in. Back in Lavender Menace I picked up a magazine called *On our Backs* which I knew was lesbian pornography/erotica. I opened it up on a picture of lesbian S/M and thought, 'Yeuch, if that's lesbian sex I don't want it' and put it back. From that I've decided that I'm against lesbian S/M.

I've done a lot of rationalizing from that gut reaction. I still think S/M is something we all do to varying degrees some of the time, but it's something I'm working away from. Becoming separatist has helped me to see that if there's something I don't like in the world it's not right for me to give any energy to it or to work with it in any way I can comfortably avoid, and that goes for S/M too. Hopefully, my energies are now being used to create an alternative for me and other womyn so that more and more we can free ourselves from sexism, classism, racism, homophobia, ageism, ableism and all the other 'isms', S/M and patriarchy. I see them all as the same thing really, all the ways we treat each other without respect. I know from reading *Coming to Power* that it's possible to do S/M and be really respectful to other womyn at the same time, but I think the activity itself isn't and that it's something to be worked against. But some womyn seem to see it as a really big, damning evil. I don't think of it as being any worse than so many of the other shit things in the world. As a vegan I've been hassled by a vegetarian who doesn't use aluminium pans. Maybe we all just do what we can.

I do feel empathy for womyn who need S/M for sexual expression. I empathize with the pain in them that brings it about; we all have that pain in some form. I have been very self-destructive in the past and still am sometimes. I see my separatism and working on honest relationships of all sorts with womyn to be part of me getting away from that. I still have some masochistic fantasies. In fact, when my lifestyle became less destructive I had them more so. I'd like them to stop altogether, though, and believe they will the more my life comes together. I think they came up more when it was first getting together because enough shit was out of my life for me to be able to deal with the less obvious things. I feel like it's safe for me working through these issues in my head since I can change and grow and move on as soon as I'm ready. Apart from the fact that acting them out wouldn't give me any pleasure I also would be tied to them, they would be part of my reality if shared with someone else and it'd be harder to let go of them. That's why when womyn say they're into S/M therapy I don't think it's a very good way of doing it.

I do think power imbalance is a form of S/M, though I'm not sure it's always mild and I believe that imbalance must be confronted for a relationship to continue as, sooner or later, someone stops getting what they need from it, usually the 'weak' one. I think most relationships have inherent power differences, but in good ones the differences are small and both womyn have areas where they have more power. If, at the same time, you're both working on not wielding your power over the other, well, you've got it made!

TANYA

I have very mixed feelings about the issue of lesbian sadomasochism. I feel that there should be a ban on the use of the swastika and badges with express racist or sexist slogans because these represent an evil ideology which destroyed and continues to destroy the people of the world. I feel that the rest of S/M paraphernalia is more to do with western punk youth culture than with Hitler's Germany or the National Front although, of course, there is some overlap. I feel that it is the intent of clothing and not clothing itself that is important. I find the idea of banning Doc Martens and leather jackets ludicrous and dangerously proscriptive, as well as degrading and belittling to the would-be wearer. We must be allowed some freedom of expression in our clothing as in everything else. What's the point of struggling for gay rights if we're repressed to that minutely detailed extent within the gay community itself? There is a growing 'thought police' mentality within the lesbian and feminist movement that censors opinions, words and now clothing. It must be resisted, though with sensitivity for the issues involved.

I have never particularly been the victim of physical violence; I dislike it intensely. I feel that S/M is not so much immoral as a symptom of our world and times. I certainly would not condone violence against S/M practitioners as it would be too reminiscent of the gay-bashing we could all fall victim to. The woman from Leeds who entered Chain Reaction with a crowbar was a particularly frightening element of the anti-S/M lobby. I think this was absolutely disgraceful.

The trouble with S/M is that one is never told what it involves. The same goes for 'vanilla sex'. I don't have a clue what my lesbian friends get up to in bed, which probably goes to show why the S/M lobby is so keen to air a subject which feminist lesbians have, puritanically, been repressing. I sometimes think that S/M must just be a reaction to the playing-down of sex and sexuality on the part of radical feminism.

I have a very warm and trusting relationship with my lover so that, although we have hit each other in anger on some occasions and we do indulge in some rough horseplay, I wouldn't particularly want to ritualize the violence and integrate it into our relationship, as I would find it alienating. Our relationship involves a power struggle, naturally, but I don't think this can be compared with a cultural localized western practice. But, obviously, people have been beating and torturing each other since the beginning of the world. I imagine that many people, gay and straight, young and old, male and female, practise S/M in their sex lives, but they don't wear the gear of a lesbian youth punk subculture. The human mind is very shadowy and complex, but people like the anti-S/M lobby are a bit frightened of this fact and they therefore scapegoat the tiny minority of S/M dykes who are fairly young, marginal, and definitely wield no real power in the world. Yet they provoke strong emotions of hatred.

There are a lot of problems and injustices in the world. I would like people to address the important things and not something which is, as far as I can see, a fashion, a youth reaction, an expression of the 'west'. Only in the west, where living standards are relatively high and torture and brutality relatively unknown, could there emerge S/M as a fashion and a sexual practice. In other parts of the world cruelty and torture is not a matter of sexual choice.

ANNA

The thing that has upset me the most about the S/M debate is the fighting between women that I know and love. Living in London and being a feminist lesbian it's impossible not to know when something as awful as this is going on. But then, it's not just the S/M debate that seems to bring out viciousness in some women. I've been very distressed at the glee some women feel or appear to feel when there's an opportunity to criticize other women. It seems impossible for us to respect each other and hold different views. I wonder if this is because, though London is huge, feminists in London are often rather parochial. Is this due to our imperial past?

I do think heavy S/M is bad. I do believe it to be a reflection of male domination that exists in the male world we live in. I do believe that the costume of S/M is fascist in origins and that it encourages a fascist presence in a culture that is already pretty right-wing. I am Jewish. I listened to my father scream in his nightmares in terror that the Nazis were going to get him, more nights than I can remember. But actually I think dog collars and chains and whips and all that stuff are, after the initial shock, rather more stupid than threatening. and of course a lot, not all, of the wearers haven't the faintest idea of Jewish and Nazi history. Perhaps that's too generous.

I must say that I shrink from the sight of a Union Jack. But that's as much to do with England's history as it is that I know the wearer is probably a fascist. Okay, let's have a dress code, but who is going to enforce it? I remember a meeting in 1985, I think, when a group of women met the woman who used to run a well known bar. She was anxious to discuss the workings of such a code for her bar. The outcome was that a large number of the women there said it would be her job to enforce it. Great; can you see it? Running the bar till all hours and getting your head stoved in every week because it was your job to see no one wore a dog collar. The final decision was that we would all be ready to share the responsibility. But I don't think anyone ever did very much. For me the situation was the usual one: a group of women ready to criticize, but not ready to do any work.

I think a lot of us use a power imbalance to handle relationships. I know many relationships like that. I'm sure that most lesbians enjoy, for example, being constrained a little during lovemaking, or being held down. Vigour is not confined to those who practise S/M. I must make a distinction, however, between such 'normal' practices and the terrifying practices of cutting, etc.

And, yes, I do have fantasies that could, I think, be described by the purists as being slightly S/M in overtone. I suppose you want the details . . . eh? Okay, it's pretty mild, so no need to get worried. I have this fantasy where I'm in the steam-baths and I'm slumped over one of those old-fashioned cage-like showers with the water going full blast, and some nameless woman is making love to me, the point being that I can't move from this metal structure. Then, once, when I was involved with a very scruffy jeans-and-trainers type woman, in a rather delightful fantasy I dressed her in a very tight Victorian corset/basque and made love to her while she was at my mercy.

In theory, aren't all fantasies involving another person, using that person without her knowledge, therefore S/M in their power imbalance? Maybe I'm lucky, I've never been turned on by rape or pain. I did once have a lover who said she was into S/M and once, to be obliging, I let her trail a leather thong all over me, but I think I yawned. Anyway, that was the beginning of the end of that relationship.

Finally, may I relate a sad little tale? I was in the Fallen Angel on a rare hot summer evening last year when a dear young friend asked me if she could ask me something in confidence. I said, 'Sure' and prepared myself – for what? Had she gone back to men and wanted to know about contraception? Had she stolen something in a moment of temptation? No. Her question was, had I read *Coming to Power*, and what did I think of it? We spent the evening talking a little about the book, but mainly about the current situation which made her come to me in secret. I was, she said, the only person she knew she could discuss it with. And she was immensely popular with an enormous circle of friends.

9

Community

INGRID

Clause 28 has made a lot of noise in British society and we, as lesbians and gay men, have got a lot of mileage out of being visible as a group or groups. I joined OLGA at one stage and went to an AGM but was so miserable at all the men behaving just like straight men, hogging space and so on, that I subsequently left the organization. I have also made the decision that I don't spend time with men unless I'm paid for it. This means, at work, teaching music, nothing else!

Although I know quite a lot of really nice gay men, I am confused and upset by some aspects of their lifestyle. I just read a book called *Anticlimax* by Sheila Jefferys. In it are detailed a lot of sexual practices which I find extremely abhorrent. I can't believe that any of my gay male acquaintances indulge in such things, but it adds to the increasing feeling I have that lesbians are not gay in the same way that gay men are. We're a different species or something. There are a lot of dykes out there who got to where they're at by the same route as I did, and it has got to do with separating from men in a big way. Nevertheless, I would acknowledge wholeheartedly that gay men are oppressed. Society at large despises us all as being unnatural, whereas I never felt so natural in all my life! This does not, however, make it any easier to work with men of any persuasion. Gay men have all the privilege conferred as a result of biological difference that straight men do. And I'm quite sure that, had the AIDS virus gotten into the lesbian community, gay men would not have been as supportive of us as we are of them. I don't mind talking about AIDS. I think it is an awful thing and something we must all care

about and fight. We as lesbians are a very low-risk group of the
population but I do feel supportive of gay men around that issue,
because it is not them that are really spreading it but the intravenous drug-user population, as far as I am aware.

I am glad for women-only spaces. They are extremely important and I find it very oppressive when they are invaded by
transsexuals, who are a surgical construct in my opinion. I think
that these poor people should be helped to confront their homosexuality, which seems to be what their problem is, and, heaven
knows, they do face awful difficulties. But I don't want male-to-
female transsexuals in women's spaces, no way! They are men.

Of course, as a lesbian, I am oppressed by the patriarchy,
doubly so, as a woman and as a lesbian who rejects the society
of men in general.

I really don't think that lesbians and gay men can work together
very effectively until the men get rid of their preconceptions
about biological superiority as men, which is a great pity, but,
because of that, I am putting all my energy into women right
now and, until things change, neither will I.

GRACE

When I was younger and more naive I thought a 'political lesbian'
was a lesbian who was interested in politics. I could hardly believe
it when I found out what it really meant. It seems to me it is no
different from a gay person forcing themselves to be heterosexual
for exterior reasons, like religion or the law or to gain the
approval of society. Also, there is something repellent about it;
it has the feeling of being exploitative or patronizing. What I
mean is, I would not like to be involved with a woman and find
that she was basically het but making herself a lesbian for a
political reason. That would make me feel used or, at least,
certainly put upon, as if I was a sort of accessory to her political
costume. There is no reason why a het woman can't be a feminist.
In fact, the more het feminists there are, the better, because they
are in a better position to influence het society from within than
we gays from outside. If you take the view that only a few people
are one hundred per cent gay or het, and most are somewhere
on a scale between, then I suppose a woman who is around the
middle of the scale can choose which side she leans to. But I
hope she would make the choice guided by her own preference

and knowledge of herself, not what was expected of her by others. If people are not true to themselves, they are going to be screwed up.

I usually refer to myself as a gay woman. I also refer to myself as a lesbian, but only when I don't feel I am being coerced into doing so. 'Dyke' I am not so sure about. I don't think I would use it myself from choice, but I don't object to it when used in a positive way by other gay women. It has the virtue of being short, and has a cheery, defiant feel about it which is good, but its having been used so much in a derogatory way makes it a word to think twice about. It all depends on the context. It's like 'queer'. I think the time will come when we can use these words freely without any hint of putting ourselves down, but maybe it hasn't come yet, except among friends where we all know what we mean. I really loathe deliberate mis-spellings of 'woman' and 'women'.

Of course I am a feminist. Anybody of either sex, gay or het, who has the slightest sense of justice cannot be other than a feminist. A feminist believes in the equality of the sexes, and does not judge people by their reproductive organs. A feminist does not presume to know anything else about a person on knowing that person's sex. Unfortunately, it is possible to be a lesbian without being feminist. You have to have cotton-wool between your ears, but they have.

The only exclusive lesbian group I belong to contains women with such diverse views they often seem to have nothing in common with each other, never mind with me. But then that means there's usually one or two I agree with on any topic, and a few I disagree with. I don't regard a person as an enemy because we have different opinions. I've often been staggered by the nonsense I read in lesbian publications, but I don't encounter hostility in person, because I don't go into situations where I would find it. I have too much else to do, and even if I had nothing else to do, I would rather do nothing than go to a conference which advertised no admittance to S/M or leather gear, and no discussion on these topics. And anybody who does go to such a conference ought to know what to expect and not go moaning to *The Pink Paper* afterwards. I am not an S/M or a leather person myself but I find that people who are strongly opposed to S/M and bisexuals tend to be of the rigidly authoritarian temperament which I find pretty uncongenial. And I wouldn't bother trying to reason with them because their minds are closed. I am not brave, I don't have a loud voice. I'm not good at putting my thoughts into words at short notice, and I can't conjure up screaming hysterics at will.

I haven't found assumptions being made about my politics because I'm lesbian, but I did once get into an argument with a young man who just couldn't understand that, although I was on a demonstration protesting against the racial harassment of Asian schoolchildren, I wouldn't sign his petition demanding the withdrawal of troops from Northern Ireland. He seemed to see them as a sort of package deal, rather than the two separate issues which to me they clearly were. I can well believe some people think being a lesbian is part of a package deal too.

DINA

I became a lesbian when I was nineteen and I did so completely within female circles, within a group of feminist friends. It had nothing to do with gay men and I called myself a lesbian right from the start. The word 'gay' had quite apolitical connotations for me at that time, and especially it seemed to indicate non-feminist women. That was in 1976.

Nevertheless, I was never a separatist in any sense, I was a socialist after all. Before I came out to myself I had only known one or two gay men, but after I became a lesbian I was immediately interested in gay politics. My lover and I joined a group called Socialist Homosexuals, which quickly changed its name to Socialist Lesbians and Male Homosexuals! Apart from us there were only one or two women who attended sporadically, yet about ten men. Nevertheless, they were all very politically okay men and I don't recall any actual friction, but there was the constant sense of being 'other' and of having to explain to them about lesbian perspectives. I became friends with a number of gay men then. Throughout my adult life my only male friends have been gay, but they are never close friends, they just don't rate in the same way women do for me.

I remember the big disco explosion in the late seventies and my friends and I going out and dancing a lot, sometimes in mostly gay men's clubs. Then around the time that clones first appeared, some of the gay men I knew were really eager to go off and involve themselves in an exclusively male lifestyle and politics. I remember this causing concern, not just to women, but to some other gay men. Then, a couple of years later, when the sexually free life for men was at its peak, my lesbian friends and I had many conversations about cruising, anonymous sex and the like. We wondered what we had to learn from gay men. Would we be better off if we could just go into the park across the road and have a quick fuck? The idea fascinated us, but also revealed what a huge divide there was between us and men. I think I wished we could do what they did but, at the same time, I was always sure that we had a richer emotional life, which I wouldn't have swapped. It seems ironic now that, in fact, lesbians did start to become more sexually adventurous, probably influenced by gay men, around the same time that HIV was taking hold.

I don't have absolutist views on the gender divide. You can be a separatist over some things and not over others. I see lesbians and gay men having some mutual interests – after all, we were all 'abnormal' and excluded from the family – but as having some interests which in no way concern the other. It's boring that some people still haven't realized why there's the need for women–only space and events, and I certainly object to words like 'apartheid' being used to describe that. It's constantly annoying as a woman to see gay men so completely oblivious to the fact that lesbians exist; they really do think that gay means male, and that their world is all there is. They are mostly unaware of the vibrant and complex world that lesbians move in. To some extent I don't care about that, it's not my business to try and tell them about my life. But as I have worked in various gay media projects over the years, time and again I've come up against their narrowness of vision. I would never opt out as a response to that. But I do always have lesbian projects on the boil that have nothing to do with gay men and that's where my strength comes from.

The other thing that is really striking in the difference between the two groups is how much more visible, attractive and successful gay men are than lesbians. There are many more famously gay men than women; there are all the modern singers like Boy George and so on; gay men can be comfortable with their image as trendsetters in design and fashion; lesbians are the dowdy poor relations. It is a cliché, but probably true, that it all comes down to money and power and basically gay men are better off *because they're men*. It's hard to confront that without falling into the position of being the whinger. That's why, when working in mixed groups, I prefer to get on and *do* things and, if necessary, do lesbian-orientated things, than waste time confronting the men.

So, I support some men-only or women-only political campaigns. I don't support men-only social space in mixed venues, they have enough of that already. I think we need to come together over some things. In principle, I support things like the campaign to lower the age of consent for gay men, but I would probably not devote any energy to it because there are things I need to be doing on my own behalf. But I have done work around AIDS, because I personally care about the men involved and because, on a larger level, I see an attack on gay men as an attack that concerns me. I fully support a mixed gay media because I think that if lesbians left gay men to run the gay papers, then gay men would happily go their own way, dominating all discussion of issues and questions which concern us all. For example, if Channel Four's lesbian and gay series *Out on Tuesday* had been separated, as some gay men argued it should be, then probably men would have got all the attention; they are more confident and glamorous in straight terms. But, even more annoyingly, they would have blithely gone ahead and defined the issues solely in terms of their interests. That's what's infuriating to a lesbian, to see men speaking as though they represent everyone, without realizing that, in fact, they speak only for themselves. Yet they do it again and again because they are oblivious to the existence of different groups of people.

I was never a lesbian separatist because I disagreed with that from a feminist position. But neither have I exclusively wanted to work with women, because I've always been aware of the different position I'm in from straight feminists. So my life has been a mixture of different political groups and interests, very much depending on circumstance and what the political climate is at any given moment. And my social life reflects that diversity in that I mostly mix with women friends, mostly lesbian but some straight, but at some times in my life there have been a few gay men I've been close to.

STEPH

First, let me say that I hate labels. I think that's the problem with most things, putting people in little boxes, like straitjackets, and nailing the lids shut. You can only be biased against someone or something if you've been able to label it. All labels carry a series of preconceptions. Having said that, I'll also confess to being just as prejudiced as anyone else, just as likely to label people and attach stereotypes to those labels!

I would define myself as a lesbian (most definitely) and also as a feminist, but *not* as a lesbian feminist. It's very hard to put into words what I see as a 'lesbian feminist', and why it's different. It's more a set of attitudes than a distinct character type. Separatism seems to me the end of the line of which 'lesbian feminist' is the beginning. The idea that female is better in all things, that women are *never* responsible for their actions, or lack of action, that it's always men's fault. Yes, men rape, or batter, and the like, but the issue isn't always that clear-cut. Some women do stay in destructive relationships when they don't need to, and I cannot stand the attitude that makes them the poor innocent victim. Women have to be responsible for themselves. The lesbian feminist line is that it's *always* someone else's fault, either a man or patriarchy in general. I have great arguments with friends about this!

I can't get on with separatism at all. It seems crazy in a world where the only way to survive is to work together, that some women want to cut themselves off completely. Where do you draw the line? Don't relate to men? Don't relate to women who relate to men? Don't get on a bus with a male driver? Don't eat food produced by men? It's simply impractical. And if men did the same, think of the outcry!

I once read a short story. I can't remember what it was called, who it was by, or where it appeared, but it was about an island community. Separatists bought the island and lived on it; men weren't allowed to land. Towards the end of the story they realize that outside society is shipping lesbians to the island, that they have been exiled and their paradise is a prison. I can see that happening!

I can't understand political lesbianism at all. How can you 'choose' to be a lesbian for political reasons? You either are or you aren't. It's not about rational things like choice. It's about feelings and attraction, emotion, love, lust. It's about feeling closer to women in every way, lovers, friends, companions. I could no more choose to be straight than I could flap my arms and fly to the moon, so how can a straight woman choose to be gay? I tend to think it's a way of avoiding the consequences, a sort of 'See, I'm not *really* queer, I'm just making a logical choice in an oppressive society; if society changed I'd be normal again' attitude. I didn't choose to be gay. I just am. I love being gay, mind. I love women. I love being with women. I love making love with women. I love the extra closeness I can have with women friends. I wouldn't change one iota of that, even if I could, but it wasn't a choice. I just grew up and found all my attention was directed towards women. I was never attracted to men or any particular man. It was always women. When I was younger I wasn't as pleased with my life as I am now, but that wasn't because I didn't like being gay, more that I didn't like how society felt and tried to make me feel about being gay.

I can understand women being heterosexual and later finding themselves attracted to women, even being married for twenty years before they realize, but that isn't a conscious choice, it's a realization of feelings. I don't believe there is such a thing as a true political lesbian. I think there are just women who are afraid of being labelled 'lesbian' with all the negative values society in general applies. It's funny, people are never afraid of being labelled 'straight'. People don't mind labels, only the wrong ones.

As far as my own choice of label goes, I call myself lesbian, dyke or gay woman at various times, depending on the company or the mood I'm in. I don't use homosexual because I think it puts the emphasis on sex, and although that's a very important, maybe the most important, part of being gay it's not the only part, there are a whole lot more emotions than just lust. I never use spellings like 'womon' or 'wimmin'; it annoys me. Language changes and grows but not by artificial bastardization. Language means something, words mean something. I always get angry with people who fuss about excluding 'man' from 'woman' as if it made a difference. As if 'history' had anything to do with 'his'. I've had some volatile discussions about that as well. I work on the principle that 'plumber' is far more exclusive of women than 'chairman', and it doesn't matter what they call you as long as they pay you right and give you respect!

In spite of this, I call myself feminist and, yes, I frequently

experience hostility from other lesbians as well as straight feminists, I'm afraid. I hold strong views and can be assertive, even
aggressive, about expressing them. My friends say I'm stubborn,
pig-headed and loud-mouthed. I won't tell you what others call
me! I've never been officially excluded but I've sometimes felt
excluded. I've also felt excluded by background. This is where
I'm 'classist' as well.

I might live in a cathedral town but I was born in London in
what was then a fairly rough working-class area. I've got a thick
cockney accent and, although I'm very intelligent, but not
modest, I don't always understand the big words some middle-
class feminists use. I grew up knowing strippers and barrow-
boys, prostitutes and conmen and my views on prostitution and
pornography reflect this. I used to sit in the women's group
listening to them saying how few working-class women they
knew and how they needed to attract more to the group, and
feel that they were out of touch. They'd got no idea about looking
after the four kids and getting the old man's dinner ready before
he came back from the pub . . . In some of the discussions I had
three choices: (1) carry a dictionary; (2) not understand what was
going on; (3) keep interrupting to ask, 'What does that word
mean?' Often I might have read the word but not known how
it was pronounced. 'Hegemony' was a good one, as I recall.

What does feminism mean to me? That's a hard one; it's almost
easier to define what it's not. A feminist is a woman who puts
other women first. A woman who does not believe that men and
women are unequal, who is willing to struggle for total equality
of opportunity in every sphere for all humans. Not all people are
equal, not everyone can be a brain surgeon, but a roadsweeper
is just as valuable and just as necessary and has just as much right
to a decent home, healthcare, education and so on. This means
that a feminist believes that men and women are equal, not the
same. No one ought to be daft enough to think that there are
no differences, just that the differences shouldn't count in most
things. Women are no more superior than men are. And women
ought to be responsible for themselves and not rely on others.
All humans have a right to work, all have a duty to look after
themselves, their homes and their children. A feminist ought to
believe that a woman who stands by and lets a man beat her
child to death *is* responsible for that neglect, even if she is also a
victim. Men and a patriarchal society should only be blamed for

the things they are responsible for. Most men are brought up by women. If anyone can change the way society runs it has to be the women who raise the next generation of men.

A feminist is simply someone who refuses to act as if women are second-class citizens and works to make this a reality for all women.

It is arguable that Section 28 of the Local Government Act, 1988, which proscribed the 'promotion of homosexuality' and 'pretended families' in schools and in local government-funded projects and events, has had a negligible effect. However, early in 1988, the ramifications of Clause 28 devastated the community. A virtue of mass-observation is that it freezes in time immediate reactions.

ANNA

I'm not quite sure where to start. The whole situation is so terrible and so bleak, although I'm sure there must be others like myself who have a secret feeling that our worst expectations have finally been realized. Through the past years while lesbian and gay rights have been recognized in some departments, and funded, I tried to squash the subversive thought that it couldn't last forever. But this is not something I'd say to just anyone. However, negativity apart, it's obvious this present government is potty. Look at the other inhumane legislation we're having to put up with.

I don't actually think we can talk about the government's 'intent' as if it was one body we're dealing with. The government is composed (some would say decomposed!) of any number of individuals. If we understand this then it's easy to see how malice and ignorance and even good, though misguided, intention can go hand-in-hand. Many government officials have far too many issues to handle, so when it comes to educating themselves out of homophobia they obviously don't have the motivation to start with nor the time, even if they thought it worthwhile. Therefore, I'm sure that many of them really believe there's no censorship or denial of human rights involved. What they haven't foreseen is that, together with the homophobia, which is always denied, of the individuals on local councils plus the pressure from government on those same local councillors to cut spending, the first out will always, in such situations, be lesbians and gays.

I come back to my original subversion. Maybe it's safer like

this. If a majority of heterosexuals feel threatened we're bound
to suffer. Maybe we'll suffer less back in the closet. Dear me,
this is dreadful . . . do I really mean this? I suppose what I do
mean is that I'm not willing to die for this cause. And I guess I
believe it could come to that.

Nazi Germany? Yes, maybe. History never repeats itself
exactly, does it? I don't really want to think about it. I'm half
Jewish and I know those stories. I've had a metaphorical suitcase
packed for years. Maybe gays and lesbians will never have real
parity in the world until heterosexuals do to them what was done
to the Jews. Still negative.

More realistically, I can say that I've been a teacher on and off
between 1968 and 1986. In that time and in different London
boroughs I've never seen any evidence of the promotion of homosexuality. Obviously, it has been contrariwise, the promotion of
heterosexuality and marriage, never even a suggestion that a
young woman might find a life without marriage. I'm sure the
so-called promotion was merely some idealistic souls trying to
combat prejudice and bigotry. It's interesting, isn't it, that people
who would fall over backwards rather than be seen as racist don't
mind at all making offensive remarks and so-called jokes about
'queers'. This happens everywhere, of course, not just in schools.

As for the 'pretended' family relationship, I feel this is the
tragic nub of the matter. A lesbian with a child, especially if the
child was born through A.I.D., hits at the heart of the patriarchy.
Such a relationship must be denied if male power is to continue.
Of course the word 'pretended' is an insult, unless such women
and men are excused the payment of rates and taxes and so
forth which, somehow, don't seem very much pretend. How can
anyone 'pretend'? A family is a family. A woman who looks
after a child is the child's family. After all, institutions like the
Dr Barnardo's Homes refer to themselves as families of the
children they care for, so why not a woman who is a lesbian?
Better a nice safe home with a lesbian for a mother than a so-
called family where children are raped and battered by parents.

As for the end . . . I can't see it. Our struggles could peter
out. After all, we only have so much energy and time and money.
I think the clause has repoliticized us a little. Also, it's brought
us to the attention of some liberals who denied homophobia as
paranoia. Now they can see what we were talking about. And I
think it could get harder for us. Thatcherism isn't dead by a long

way. And the other parties are hardly likely to feel that success is going to be found supporting us. We have to do it ourselves. Personally, I couldn't face violence. But I'd understand those who could. I'm trying to speak up more for our cause. We're between a rock and a hard place.

Three years later, Clause 25 of the Criminal Justice Bill sought to stiffen the penalties for several crimes with which gay men are frequently charged and was seen as the precursor to the recriminalization of male homosexuality. Concurrently Paragraph 16 of the Department of Health's guidelines on the placing of children with foster parents included the assertion that ' "equal rights" and "gay rights" policies have no place in fostering services'. At the end of 1989 an Old Bailey judge sentenced eight men to up to four and a half years in prison for consensual S/M sex sessions, and related offences.

MIRANDA

1988 is currently and will probably remain one of the most important years of my life. This is mainly to do with the publication of Clause 28 of the Local Government Bill and the tremendous response to it. In retrospect, my sexuality and its effect on my life had been a very personal affair, and my main concerns like most other lesbians and gays revolved around coming out and how to do it!

Clause 28 seemed to mark the beginning of my political awareness relating to homosexuality and I threw myself into campaigning on the streets and among my friends and colleagues. I was disgusted at the implications of the clause although the ambiguity of the wording and the degree to which it would be adhered to meant it was very much an unknown quantity. No real information or statistics have been collated, to my knowledge, or could be to measure the effect of the legislation but the idea was clearly homophobic and discriminatory.

The strength of feeling at the public marches and demonstrations I attended in Manchester, Leeds and London was incredibly supportive and exhilarating and certainly appeared to make those people around take notice. Many interpretations of how the clause would affect us, our children, families and friends were on offer, but people around me seemed more concerned at the idea and the prevention of it rather than assessing possible, potential damage.

Three years later I still feel it was worthwhile even though the bill passed into law. For a few months I checked my local libraries to see if the token half-dozen or so gay books were still there. No change. The town I live in boasts, as do most Labour-run councils, an equal opportunities policy, but has never included 'sexual orientation'. My career is in social work and within my immediate circle of colleagues and clients there has been no noticeable change in attitudes and working practice. However, lately, a few of my friends have started teacher training courses on which there is a compulsory Equal Opportunities module. All have told me they have received no tutoring on homosexuality and related issues, and believe this has to be because of Clause 28. Although I have experienced few ways in which the clause has compromised the community, I'm sure it has fuelled homophobic feeling and I believe people must organize to reject any discriminatory legislation.

Clause 25 and Paragraph 16 are further examples of the government's homophobic, heterosexist attitude. Clause 25 is incredible in that the linkage of gay sex and child abuse is totally unfounded and dangerous, reinforcing the belief that child sex abuse doesn't happen in 'normal', 'decent' families, when the vast majority of it does. It makes me very angry to think that the abuse and oppression that women and children suffer is being blamed on a section of the community almost devoid of responsibility. This government will go to such lengths to find scapegoats in protecting the precious 'family life' that it ignores the facts.

The evolution of Paragraph 16 seems like a natural progression in the thinking of the government implementing its big blue-rinse over the 'normal' majority! I know of some lesbians who accept lesbianism and motherhood as an either/or choice. Like Clause 28, the response to Clause 25 and Paragraph 16 has been substantial and not only from lesbians and gays but from socialists too. I have no doubt that, if the police utilize the new law to the full, then the judges who are, in the main, male, white, hetero and over sixty will have no hesitation in sentencing.

VANESSA

I am feeling quite upset about the environmental damage in the Gulf, experiencing a sense of powerlessness in the face of patriarchal institutions such as government and army and the like, simply doing as they like, regardless of public opinion. Poll tax summonsing, no money in the NHS, ordinary people deprived of the treatment they need because it is 'too expensive', worrying about the implication of this for people with AIDS, especially gay and lesbian people with AIDS.

Section 28 has stopped my local community from getting any direct funding for the lesbian and gay centre we would like to open. The local council is Labour but still homophobic (or should that read 'Labour and homophobic'?) and yet it has had some good galvanizing effects. Every cliché has a pink lining.

As for Clause 25, I am disgusted but not surprised by it. This government would introduce aversion therapy if they thought they had half a chance of getting away with it. The police, of course, won't object. It's much easier to catch gay men 'at it' than rapists and paedophiles, isn't it? I am very glad to see the elements concerning rape and sex with children going into Clause 25, but not happy that they are lumped in with gay matters. But then, to nice straight Conservative men, we're all sick criminals, aren't we?

Paragraph 16 may mean that some self-censoring gay couples don't put themselves forward as foster parents, but I'm pleased to see that some do challenge it. Quite why, I'm not sure. I've always thought that being a lesbian was a great excuse for avoiding maternity. I hate and loathe the way women are expected to subsume their identity with the sacred confines of motherhood. Snails have it sussed: they deposit their eggs under a rock and leave. Besides, the world is over-populated as it is, so why exacerbate the problem? But this is a digression from fostering. Sorry!

I feel the S/M trial certainly was an attack on homosexuals, and is yet another aspect of anti-gay institutional prejudice. But I think those blokes were extremely stupid to send videos through the post. Of course, straight people find gay and lesbian S/M repellent; it constitutes too much of a threat to their narrow notions of what sex is about. Straight people are often boring in bed because they castrate sex of its power and danger. I would have liked a female equivalent of 'castrate' here, but there isn't one. Malespeak for which I'm apologetic.

Community policing? – ha! ha! ha! Only in San Francisco! 'Our' police are cottage-bashers and gay pub-raiders. My opinion of the police is pretty low and it's only the fact that one of my friends is a dyke cop which prevents me from being totally anti. Haven't done too well on the London gay murders, have they?

A regularly sought day-diary addresses the way observers spend the last Saturday in June, Pride Day, whether or not their activities that day are affected explicitly by their sexuality.

MARGE

It's 27 June 1987 and here is my hourly diary.

Stayed at a friend's luxury flat the night before and woke at about 9 a.m. Got up, went to the kitchen and had an illicit sandwich. Bread – white – mayonnaise and a hot chunk of delicious sausages. And I haven't finished yet. Cereal, twice, with milk. I was hungry. I sat watching the repeat performance of *Lizzie's Pictures* on the video. This is a treat for me. I sat there on my own having a good cry over it. Great.

10 a.m. Watched *The Hitch-Hiker's Guide to the Galaxy* on video too. Afterwards I ran a bath and put on Joan Armatrading on the hi-fi. Got in the bath. Aaaaah.

11 a.m. By now I'm clearing up the debris from the night before, leaving the flat tidy for my mate. There was reams of it. I feed the miserable half-wild cat. Phoned Robert, arranged to meet in Covent Garden at 1.30 p.m.

12 p.m. Still fucking tidying up. Putting on the answering machine. Pack my bag and I'm off. Cycling towards Holloway Road.

1 p.m. In 'Sister Write' buying cards. Very relaxed in there. Came out of shop. Cycled two hundred yards down road. Nearly collided with idiot who walked out on the zebra crossing right in front of me. Steered round him. He saw me. I saw him. He stopped. I carried on. Next minute flagged down by an unmarked navy-blue car. Fuck the Bill. Did I know that pedestrians had precedence at pelican crossings? Did I always ride through crossings, Madam, blah, blah. Authority, Authority. I am a nasty overbearing shit. I stood up to him. I wasn't going to be harassed

by him. He said he'd book me. Twelve pounds with two weeks
to pay. I said it was petty, the man had one foot off the crossing.
After much wrangling from me he let me off. I don't think he
was on duty.

2–4 p.m. Arrived late, chatted, went to shops, the pub and walked
down to the Strand and bumped into the Gay Parade March
which I had decided not to go to. Robert and I stood watching
the passing parade and I bumped into old friends and old lovers.
I eventually persuaded Robert to join the march and we arrived
in Jubilee Gardens jubilant.

4 p.m. The music was good with the exception of Bronski Beat.
Crap.

5 p.m. Went to beer tent, drank, sat down. I admired some
woman's outfit from afar. As well as the woman. Quietly.

6 p.m. Looked at various stalls. Queued for the toilet. Watching
the drunken lesbians and gays stumble past.

7 p.m. On the way home bump into the dreaded mother of my
three-year-not-very-certain lover, who doesn't like me. Surprise,
surprise. Hellos exchanged. Get home, ring my not-very-definite
lover, who sounds a bit depressed.

8 p.m. Potter about in flat. Flatmate arrives back drunk. She has
slept in my bed with her lover last night. I'm very pissed off.
Flatmate can't stand up straight.

9 p.m. Get ready to go out. Flatmate makes pass at me, asks to
sleep in my bed again. I'm furious, but there is no point hassling
with a person when she's drunk. The answer is no. I leave for
work. Buy some food. Arrive ready to babysit.

10 p.m. Lesley has just put Adam to bed. The two of them have
just arrived from Italy. We chat and eventually she leaves with
her boyfriend. I relax in front of the TV with my crisps and
brew and watch Germaine Greer.

11 p.m. Get into bed and lying there dream of my lover while
listening to smoochy music . . .

VI

Midnight. Arrived home after a birthday celebration at a gay club
in Luton. I hadn't enjoyed the club much, my first visit. Very
young clientele, very 'posey' and a not very friendly atmosphere.
Cabaret artist did a couple of what I considered very offensive
drag spots, one of which was sexually explicit and of the lowest

lavatorial humour. Interesting to note he didn't get too big a response from the audience. Didn't feel his material was suitable for a mixed gay audience. My friend Rita and her brother Tom, the birthday boy, wanted to leave early, partly because Rita was dashing home to meet her new lover and Tom because he's driving up to London later.

12.30 a.m. Feeling very headachey and lethargic, also vaguely queasy. Have only consumed two pints of orange and lemonade, but on reflection realize I've also had very little to eat today, toast and marmalade for breakfast, cucumber and mayonnaise on a roll at lunchtime, three crumpets with margarine for tea. Let the dog out for a pee. Look anxiously at the sky feeling spots of rain. Quite a breeze too which will make carrying the Lesbian Line banner difficult.

12.35 a.m. Warm bath makes me feel dizzy and hot. Feeling anxious about the morning. Am I going to be able to travel feeling like this? Notice my hands are still slightly pink from the cyclamen coloured Crazy Colour I put on my hair yesterday. Got into bed accompanied by my two four-month-old demolition experts (kittens!), Skye and Mandela, who insist on playing like it's the middle of the afternoon. Feel really uncomfortable and my head is pounding.

2.30 a.m. Woken by violent urge to vomit; get to the bathroom just in time. Feel violently ill and fragile like I can hardly stand up . . . wish there was someone here; it's very lonely being ill alone. Look at myself in the bathroom mirror. Face very pale and my hair looks quite shocking in contrast. The kittens and the dog sit in an interested row watching me on my knees at the loo as another wave of nausea hits me.

2.45 a.m. Back in bed with a hot-water bottle and two paracetamol. Don't usually take drugs at all but am so anxious to be better by the morning. Lie feeling cold and shakey. Can't get comfortable. Feel too grotty to be amused by the kittens who begin leaping on and off the bed. The dog also wakes up and stands, everything wagging, looking expectantly at me. I tell him to lie down and he goes back to sentry duty at the hall door.

3.30 a.m. Get up after tossing and turning and being unable to sleep to once again be sick and feel frail and giddy in the bathroom. Look out of the living-room window. All quiet outside, still drizzling with a light breeze. Make a cup of tea then find it makes me nauseous so throw it down the sink. Assure the kittens it is definitely not yet time for breakfast. Crawl back to bed. Now feel too hot with hot-water bottle and summer-weight duvet. Head still pounding and eyes and neck feeling achey and sore.

5.30 a.m. Woken by kitten jumping on my head. Realize I've had a couple of hours sleep. Sit up and decide it's more comfortable lying down. Is it a bug or a migraine? Whatever it is, I wish it would go away. Why did it have to ruin today of all days? On another trip to the bathroom I admire my waistcoat, resplendent with twenty badges – Dykes OK, Pride 90, Lesbians Rule, Sanctions Now, AA Freedom for South Africa, our local Lesbian and Gay Switchboard, etc. – hanging all ready to be worn later. Make another cup of tea and manage to drink half of it before feeling sick . . .

5.45 a.m. Back in bed thinking about how much my head hurts. Also about all the lesbian and gay friends I'm hoping to see later, excited and full of anticipation, slightly sad remembering that I'll be on my own this year as my last relationship broke up a month ago, wondering if I'll see Tilly and her new lover and how I'll feel if I do. Realizing part of me feels quite cynical in that I'm aware that so many lesbians there will be avoiding and not speaking to other lesbians there. Sisterhood? Then I reflect on the fun and cooperation that has existed among the group I belong to preparing for the march: badge-making, banner-making, both activities involving several new women. Must get some sleep. Pray for healing.

7.20 a.m. Awake again and this time with an urgent need to empty my bowels. All I need. The headache is still there and I feel hot, dizzy and shakey. Stagger back to bed after taking two more paracetamol. Animals standing looking expectant force me up again. I figure if I give them breakfast they'll possibly settle down and give me some peace. Put on trousers and trainers and a jacket over my T-shirt to stagger downstairs to take the dog for a pee. Feel really frail and can't wait to get back to bed.

8.05 a.m. The phone rings and it's my friend Alison who is sharing the car with Toni and Shirley to go up to Pride. She's recovering from a bad nervous breakdown and her sense of timing and events are still somewhat confused. I explain we won't be picking her up until 10.45. Tell her how ill I'm feeling and that I'm not sure I can make the journey. She's disappointed and suggests I try to sleep for an hour or so . . .

8.15 a.m. Postman drops off instruction manual for a Gallup Poll I'm doing next weekend. Can't face looking at it at the moment. It's sunny and bright. My eyes are hurting so I close the curtains and get back into bed.

9.10 a.m. Dozing and sweating. Another lesbian rings wanting to know the arrangements for those going up by train. I'm coordinating. I give her all the details but tell her not to expect me. She's really surprised as I've been so active in the arrangements and also encouraged her and several others to go this year. I explain my boring list of symptoms. She's suitably sympathetic. Beginning to feel really sorry for myself. I don't want to be left behind.

9.30 a.m. Two more lesbians ring for times. Toni rings and is really upset to hear I'm ill, tries to suggest what to do. Can hardly stand up at the moment so cut her short and go back to bed.

10.15 a.m. Toni rings again to confirm that I'm not going. Feeling really disappointed. Assures me she'll have me with her in spirit and will tell me all about it on Monday. Not much consolation as I stagger back to bed feeling very lonely and disappointed.

11 a.m. Dying, and wondering why my neighbour had to choose this very morning to mend his car with much crashing and banging accompanied by loud transistor music right under my bedroom window! The phone rings again. Another lesbian I met for the first time this week who was undecided whether to go on the march has made up her mind to go. If she can get to Alison's within the next ten minutes she can have my place in the car . . .

11.10 a.m. Take the dog out for another pee. Back to bed.

2.30 p.m. Actually managed to sleep all this time. Still feel lousy. Reflecting that the march will have started by now, wishing I was there, seeing a parade of all my favourite lesbians and gay men going past in my head, wishing I'd lent Toni the whistle I was going to take with me. Hope there won't be any trouble from the National Front or other yobs. Remembering the amazing strength of feeling, being part of the gay community. Us in the majority for once. Would it have been a booster for me, having been feeling cynical and disillusioned with the scene lately, lots of dissension and strife going on among the 'straight' lesbians and the 'feminists' locally. Drifting off again . . .

CHRIS

On Pride day, 29 June 1991, I woke up at my lover's flat at 8.15 a.m. when the alarm went off. After a brief cuddle I got out of bed despite her protestations; I knew that if we got into any serious cuddling we would probably be late and I hate being rushed in the morning. We got dressed in our identical outfits – white Pride T-shirts, blue jeans, black Doc Marten boots (carefully polished the night before), studded leather wristbands and black leather jackets. I had breakfast, toast, but she didn't as anything more than a cup of coffee (instant Nescafé – very right off!) upsets her tummy.

At 9.15 our taxi arrived and took us to the station and, after I had bought my ticket, we got the Intercity to London. On the train we sat gay-spotting and met a couple of fellow Gaysoc people. A friend of my lover's appeared and sat with us and on the way down we talked about our jobs, the local gay scene and speculated as to what Pride would be like.

Two hours later we arrived at St Pancras and took the tube to Temple station. We couldn't find any toilets there and had to walk all the way to Embankment where a long queue of lesbians waited at the public toilet. By the time we had walked back to Temple my legs were starting to shake and we picked up one of the wheelchairs which the Pride committee had laid on. I have M.E. and can't walk very far. This was the first time since my illness began four months ago that I had had to rely on a wheelchair and it felt like a big giving-up of control.

My lover started wheeling me down the pavement towards the front of the march and we passed pink balloons, people in drag, groups of lesbians and gays with banners, and floats driving up and down, all adding to the general air of excitement. There were also several phalanxes of policemen, grim-faced and determined not to enjoy themselves, which lent a rather sinister air to the proceedings. Several people gave us embarrassed smiles or made patronizing remarks and I felt very conspicuous. A man holding a bunch of whistles said to me, 'Here you are, dear, have a free whistle from Outrage'.

Soon the march started off with much cheering and blowing of whistles and soon people were lining the route as we waved and blew our whistles to them. Cars passing by on the other side of the road who hooted were greeted with cheers and more whistles blowing. After a while we hung back to wait for the S/M Gays' banner to go by and, as we spotted it, we caught up and marched with them. Much to our surprise and delight, one of the group asked if we were interested in S/M and gave us a leaflet about their tenth birthday celebrations which were coming up. People on the march shouted slogans like, 'We're here, we're queer, and we're not going shopping' and there was an interesting selection of T-shirts on display, including 'Queer as fuck' and 'Trade entrance at rear'.

Eventually we arrived at Kennington Park and decided to have a look round the stalls. My lover found it heavy going as the ground was very soggy and uneven. We ran into several people we knew who didn't know about my M.E. and who reacted in various ways. One looked appalled but didn't say anything about it, another asked if I had hurt my foot and one asked what it was and seemed happy and comfortable talking about it. We also ran into the two bisexual people I live with and our baby. She sat on my knee in the chair and we talked about my pushchair and hers and looked through the publications in my bag. We went to the Clone Zone stall to get me a Muir cap and some handcuffs. I had to get out of my chair as nobody would get out of my way to let me get close to the stall in the wheelchair. We also looked at Della Grace's book *Love Bites* and decided that there were a few good pictures in it but not enough to justify buying it.

My lover was getting worn out by this time so we sat down and had some Veggieburgers and a rest. It was nearly 7 p.m. by this time so I returned my wheelchair and we went to the main stage to watch Nomad. They came on after a couple of other acts and did a short, but brilliant, set. When they had finished we were both very tired and decided to go home.

We made our way to the tube station, which was packed with gay people, and met a couple of friends we had seen earlier. Our carriage was full of gays who, at one point, burst into a communal chorus of 'I am what I am'. We arrived at St Pancras, by which time I was having a hard job coping with the numerous stairs. We finally made it on to the late train and sat talking about being gay in a het world and how to cope. When we got home we chatted briefly about our day before falling exhausted into bed and rapidly to sleep.

RUTH

The first gay bar I ever went to was an accidental event. I was seventeen and besotted with one of my best friends at school. We'd been out together for the evening and on the way home decided to stop for a drink. Although it was a fairly local pub, neither of us had ever been in it before. We'd bought our drinks and were sitting down when I started to look round, the way one often does in a strange pub. It was then that I noticed that nearly all the other drinkers were men and that, for the most part, they seemed to be in couples. I realized immediately that it must be a gay pub and felt strangely elated. At seventeen I'd had only straight relationships although I was increasingly aware that it was women I felt attracted to and wanted to be with. The friend I was with that night was straight and so I couldn't share my feelings of joy with her at having found a gay pub. It was to be over two years before I went to another gay pub, but at least then it was a conscious choice.

At nineteen I was working and living in London and very gradually coming out to myself and to a few other people I trusted. I knew only two lesbians then and one night they took me along to Gateways. I'd seen the bar featured in the film of *The Killing of Sister George* but somehow it had seemed bigger in the film. I remember we had to go through a door on the street and then down some steps to another door where we were vetted, signed in, and then finally allowed inside. It was dark and smoky and I don't suppose there were more than thirty people inside. I felt rather cheated; I think I thought it would be filled to the gills with women drinking, dancing and, of course, all snogging furiously. Instead, it seemed to be full of women, mostly in their thirties, sitting around chatting or propping up the bar. I can only remember one woman clearly from that evening. She was serving behind the bar and must have been in her fifties. She had close-cropped grey hair, was smoking and, to me, she looked like the butchest dyke I could imagine. I never went back again.

ROSEMARY

Bars have played very little part in my life. I was brought up abroad where women did not go to bars much. In Britain I have been to a few pubs with my mate, encouraged to go there by lesgay friends. Ugh. Noisy, smoky, conversation impossible. Cannot understand why anyone goes to pubs. I can't remember the first pub I went to which is odd as I've been to so few. One of them was supposed to be a gay pub and our lesgay campaigning group met there in a back room for a while. Then the pub went het rather nastily. 'Fuck off, fairy,' was said over the phone to a member trying to book the room. The main pub bit was mainly het, I suppose, dull old men sitting about, as far as I can recall. I couldn't understand why, when we met later in a nice spacious clean library room, the rest of the group missed their grotty pub. Two members stopped coming, they would miss their drink. When I suggested they could bring tins of lager with them to the meetings the others stared at me as if I had said the *most peculiar thing*. Then they tried holding the meetings in a public bar. I couldn't believe it, trying to speak above the noise of music and other people shouting. One member said he preferred to drink in pubs because he did not believe in drinking at home. I noticed that when we had evening meetings in a left-wing bookshop the business had to be galloped through in order to have time for that drink in the noisy stuffy pub en route home. Needless to say, I never joined them in this treat. The Brit's attachment to pubs is to me the strangest national characteristic. They all seem better at lip-reading than I am; I suspect they have to be if they spend so much time in noise-polluted pubs.

When I was first interested in meeting other lesbians and lesbian groups, feeling that my mate and I were very cut off from making lesbian friends, most of the scene, especially lesbian, was inaccessible for disabled people. At that time I longed to go to the big lesbian meetings which were held in a room above a pub, where there were speakers and special interest nights, poetry readings and so on, as well as the beer. I could not go because of lack of access. Now, because I have some noise-free smoke-free socials to go to, I wouldn't go to the main lesbian gatherings if I was paid to, and they *still* meet in inaccessible rooms above pubs, the antediluvian dears.

GRACE

What's in a name? Logically, nothing, but I resent the current fashion of sticking 'lesbian and' in front of 'gay' whenever it appears. I object to waste of time, space and energy, and insistence on these redundant syllables wastes all three. More seriously, I dislike it because it removes gay women from the mainstream and relegates us to a sort of appendage ('lesbian and') which can be readily chopped off. I like the word 'gay' because it is short and because it annoys blimpish hets who deplore the loss of that 'pleasant little word' and I do not agree to give it up to the exclusive use of men. Gay is me. Lesbian is me too, but as a subdivision within gay, not an alternative to it. Analogy: I am a Scot, I am also a Glaswegian. Sometimes I think of myself as the one, sometimes the other, depending on the context, but to talk about 'Glaswegians and Scots' would be nonsense.

'Pride March' is a spineless cop-out. I make a point of always referring to the Gay Pride March, Gay Pride Week, the Gay Centre and Gay Switchboard. One of the gay groups to which I belong has kept its original name. Despite not having tacked 'lesbian and' on to our name we have a good proportion of women active and prominent within the group.

I don't like the existence of women-only space in gay centres and at rallies. I think such places and events should be wholly open to all gay people. It follows that I would not like black-only or disabled-only, or even Scots-only spaces. An entirely separate lesbian centre is a slightly different matter. If a category of people choose to organize themselves and establish their own centre and exclude all others then, while I might wish they didn't, I have to admit they must have the freedom to do so. I belong to a women-only group which was formed to serve the interests of a particular section of gay women. We decided from the outset that it had to be women only, because the small collective that runs the group would not have the time or resources to cope with the numbers if men were admitted. We have had men join the group pretending to be women. One actually attended a meeting, sitting there with his moustache on asking us how we knew he *wasn't* a woman. We feel angry at this deception and expel these men when we find them. We are not so unanimous on the subject of transsexuals. I am for regarding them as women if they so regard themselves, other members are not. We have no set policy on transsexuals and tend to assess them on an individual basis. If a man were to enter the women-only space at, for instance, the Gay Centre, I would suspect his motives, that he was looking for trouble. So I would ignore him, in the belief that if someone is looking for trouble, nothing upsets him so much as not getting it.

I wouldn't like to see men-only space at the Gay Centre. In effect, it is there already when there are meetings of men-only groups, but I would resent seeing part of the building devoted to men on a permanent basis. I imagine that resentment is what men feel when they see women-only space. Perhaps I am wrong in projecting my feelings on to men in that way. I haven't asked any men how they feel about women-only space. I don't think I would get an honest answer.

We do still have an oppressive patriarchal society. There have been great advances during my lifetime but there is still a long way to go and I am afraid the rate of advance is slowing down and is about to stop and even reverse under the pressure of religious fundamentalism. Gay men are part of the patriarchal oppression. I think most of them dislike women. They probably don't hate us quite as much as het men do, because they have no need of us, they just wish we didn't exist. So we have to fight them. We don't do this by separating ourselves from them, but rather by getting in there and standing up for ourselves and our right to acceptance as equals. Any little thing we do helps, even if it's only pulling them up every time they call us 'ladies' in that patronizing voice. They will do it again next week, but if we keep at it it might eventually sink in. I don't believe in giving up and retreating to a separatist ghetto which is what the misogynists would like us to do. I see no contradiction between fighting *with* gay men and *against* them; gay women have two battles. Gay men are our allies in one and our enemies in the other. This is all sweeping generalization: there are some men, gay and het, who are genuinely non-sexist. I don't believe the non-sexist men are the guilt-ridden right-on brothers who conscientiously tack 'lesbian and' on to everything and who say things like, 'We must get more women in the group' – you can practically hear them thinking, but never saying, 'then they can form a women's section and hold their own meetings and we won't have to have them at ours'. Of course, I deplore manhating in women as much as misogyny. Both are the results of mental laziness, where one cannot be bothered to find out what another person is really like, but assumes that because one knows that person's gender one therefore knows all there is to know about them. What's in a person's head is more important than what's between their legs, and I have more in common with a man who is interested in politics and books than with a woman who is interested in dancing and snooker; not that there is anything wrong with dancing or snooker, they're just not my things.

Obviously the cause must suffer from separation. It's lucky that our enemies don't know the half of the in-fighting that goes on within the gay movement, or we would lose all credibility. A few years ago an organization was formed called DAFT (Dykes and Faggots Together) which was to be for political action by gay men and women. I thought this seemed like a good idea and went along to the first meeting. The woman co-organizer went to some trouble to explain how she was all for women-only groups and activities, but there just might be a place for a bit of joint campaigning. Then the meeting spent most of its time bellyaching about Gay Conservatives and Gay Christians, and proposing letters to tell these errant brothers and sisters just what we thought of them. What a waste of time, I thought, directing our efforts against other gay people instead of against our real enemies. I didn't bother going back and I haven't heard of DAFT since. I'm afraid its name was altogether too apt. Then when something like the Gay Centre opens, one of the first things it does is get into a furious argument about what gay people it can *keep out*. What should be a unifying force becomes negative and divisive. Goddess help us. . . .

Index of authors